MONTAGUE BROWN
and BARBARA McCOOL

Active
AGING
Life Design
for Health

ACTIVE AGING: LIFE DESIGN FOR HEALTH

© 2019 by Barbara McCool and Montague (Monty) Brown

Poetry, paintings, and photographs by Monty Brown. Cover photo of desert by Monty Brown. Back cover photo by Ryan Nicholson and published by the University of Chicago Office of Gift Planning.

Thanks to Alan Goforth for his early editing and manuscript suggestions. He got us on track and back on course several times. As the first drafts began, Dr. Jeffrey Weidman provided some early editorial advice. Grammarly, an editorial application, overruled many of our errors and challenged our editorial assistants and readers. Many others were asked to review copies and offered invaluable assistance. Our neighbor Bert Bates offered invaluable suggestions for both early and later readings. Finally, our line editor furnished by Book Baby ended these debates with sound advice and insightful suggestions.

Library of Congress Control Number: 2019907393
ISBN 978-1-54398-208-4 eBook 978-1-54398-209-1

CONTENTS

DEDICATION

The love and direction of many people who have graced our lives and provided clear insights has led us to the tenet of active aging:

Our parents—Mary, Minnie, Bill, and Barney—who loved us and provided gifts of positive living, Christian values, and continuous support.

Our teachers, colleagues, children, family members, friends, and neighbors who encouraged us, taught us, and supported positive values. This work is especially dedicated to our Tucson neighbors in the Notch and our Kansas City neighbors at Bishop Spencer Place. Special thanks to all of our friends and neighbors who offered suggestions and read early drafts of some of the material.

Our health care providers and health care colleagues who continually supported us and provided research and new knowledge to light our way on the active aging journey.

Our loving animals, who have graced our lives and taught us much about living and unabashed loving.

And finally, you, the reader, who—regardless of age and physical condition—have the curiosity to learn new things and the courage to live life to its fullest.

PREFACE

As we prepared for our first retirement from 1994 to 1996, we examined the variables that would influence our lives going forward. Although we were near the average retirement age, we didn't want to retire yet; however, we were burned out and needed a long break from sustained work. So we tried to pull back from consulting and find satisfying career-type work in a place we thought would be best for us during our retirement years.

We had a good understanding of things that would help us stay active and healthy. At that time, we considered writing a book about active aging, which had long been a professional interest and personal quest of ours. We felt it was logical to consider doing this as our last professional adventure. However, writing such a book before experiencing our recommendations lacked originality; too many writers give advice without experience to back up their counsel. So instead, we continued to read, evaluate, and find practices that seemed to buttress our current aging goals. Now we can write from research on best practices as well as from direct experience.

We are health system designers, and this is a case study of our aging actively. We write from over forty years of professional life experience working in and living around modern health care. We live in the kind of retirement community that we anticipated in our system-design consulting work. This retirement community fosters the independence needed for each resident to live their dreams including a variety of physically, socially, spiritually and intellectually stimulating activities.

This is also a memoir of our aging studies and aging journey of life. This book represents our assessment of the things that have worked for us as well as those that haven't. Our experiences may help others facilitate a healthy aging lifestyle. However, each person must evaluate their own needs and responses to different approaches. Nothing works for everyone, and most things need to be tailored for each individual.

We began writing this memoir after we moved to Bishop Spencer Place, a Continuing Care Retirement Community (CCRC). Monty needed rehabilitation after heart surgery, and Barbara, who had endured the stress of caregiving and downsizing and moving our household, needed restoration as well. We knew that for recovery to work best, both of us should follow similar lifestyles.

This thinking led to an in-depth examination of factors influencing our health. Our joint program led us to research this book and redesign our lifestyles to make the most of our remaining senior years. We decided that a case study of two people seeking an ideal healthy active lifestyle might be useful to others for research and for designing their own personal aging journeys.

Over time, we realized that the science on many of the issues related to aging well is incomplete. Beliefs on what works and does not vary widely. In short, we concluded that we lack the expertise to make hard recommendations. Indeed, it is difficult for even experts to do much more than make suggestions. We are here to offer suggestions; individuals must use themselves as their own ultimate guide and decision-maker in their quest for a healthy life.

This is also a story about a real-life adventure. The story includes ideas about how to design a lifestyle using the knowledge available on many subjects relevant to healthy active aging.

We offer insights for the researcher and active ager. We provide no hard answers. Knowledge rarely comes in a form that will fit everyone. Life offers choices; some people will adapt, others not. Persistent problems—especially diseases—require self-management and much self-experimentation. Many issues have no magic solutions, but there are many options to try, and curiosity will aid in an individual's search for the right healing mix. There is wisdom in the admonition "Seek, and ye shall find."

If you intend to discover ways to become more active, to be more fit, to find and keep good friends, you will find hundreds of ideas here. However, the real challenge is that you MUST conduct research yourself. If you read something that seems feasible for you to do, stop right then and ask, **"What can I do NOW, in this present day, to move toward that goal for myself?"** It is as simple and as complicated as that. You can read a thousand books like this and make no progress. However, if you do this one simple thing each day, you can succeed in doing almost anything. We say "almost" because we have not experienced everything that a person might aspire to do. However, every time we try this method, it works: set your intention, then focus on action in the present—today—and act. Each day, repeat the process: intend an effort, pick a goal, imagine the steps, and take action. As the old slogan notes, "Just do it." We apologize in advance for often reminding ourselves of these important truths. They are hard won and ofter require us to relearn them. So for those who see this as a failure of writing, it is not just that. It is a reminder to ourselves that we must not put off what we can and should do in the present.

Two of our dear friends—Dr. Harry Prosen and Bert Bates—have written the forewords for this book. Each has a background uniquely pertinent to the subject of active aging.

Dr. Harry Prosen is an accomplished psychiatrist and professor whose lifestyle choices illustrate much of the active aging ideas presented in this book. We first met shortly after retiring to Tucson, Arizona, where both couples were at a seminar that introduced a concept for retirement—something we thought was in our near future, as did Harry. Our friendship and frequent conversation developed and continued via email and visits at Spirit Base Camp and in Milwaukee and one vacation in Canada. Many of the ideas presented in this book were the subject of our discussions over the years. We shared early chapters with Harry.

Bert Bates is an accomplished lawyer, civic leader, and ideal neighbor. He leads an exemplary life singing in his church choir and still practicing law three days a week, plus doing pro bono work in our retirement community. He eats and drinks in moderation, and at ninety-three years of age, he's still being honored for his good works; most recently, he received an honorary doctorate from the University of Missouri, as well as state- and citywide lifetime achievement awards. He has read all of the iterations of this book and encouraged us to continue on. He is an inspiration to us and many others.

Finally, we provide here a few suggestions for individuals, professionals, and public policy experts. First, individuals must take a large share of responsibility for themselves. But many individuals (and professionals) balk at the idea that they are responsible for their condition. Assigning some responsibility to the individual is sometimes frowned up and called "blaming the victim." We mean no harm in our call for self-responsibility, but without taking such responsibility, one leaves a significant curative and preventive power unexpressed. Would you rather be a victim than be cured? It is a possible choice for most. Professionals know that people who don't take better care of themselves become sicker sooner and die earlier. Public policy, however, favors solutions suggested by providers and product manufacturers; consumers don't show up early and often to lobby for their interest, which creates a void that seems unlikely to be filled. Others will sell you their products and services, but only you have the highest stake in your health. Exercise your independence and personal responsibility if you wish to enjoy the best that life has to offer.

We are not so naive as to believe that many will follow the kinds of behaviors we think work best for designing a lifestyle for excellent health as we age. We really do know how difficult it is to do this; we ourselves fail often enough to understand this issue. However, we offer our assessment in the hope that we will succeed more often than we fail and be healthier for it all. Our failings are painful but essential if we are ever to succeed. We just do our best and wish the best for everyone who tries. Go for health!

We hope you enjoy the book, but don't expect things to change in your life without daily advancing your goals via deliberate action steps taken by you.

FOREWORD

Getting old, becoming older, and the depressing term "aging" all vanish when one reads this book. Perhaps calling aging a happy time for all is unbelievable, but this book turns the pessimistic words of loss and ending into thoughts, philosophies, and actual ways for making this later stage of life not only more cheerful but also a means to gain and retain hope.

This book is about healthy aging. It's based on the autobiographies, personal searches, and answers of the authors. It also includes the expertise and ideas of other authors, young and old. It's not just a book on how to diet, exercise, and experience life and death; it's also a treatise on the life experience itself.

As you read the book, you live with the authors and the many others they have lived with and organized with, and you see the world with its many beauties. It is a book of commentaries, original lenses to observe with, and the best use of it is as a self-help book for yourself as well as those you love.

This book predicts, with great accuracy, life yet to come. The concept of life yet to come exists. Here we learn how to live it daily and into our always-challenging futures.

Harry Prosen, MD
Professor and Chair Emeritus
Department of Psychiatry, Medical School
University of Wisconsin, Milwaukee

FOREWORD

This publication is filled with information and suggestions that will be of great benefit to all but particularly to those over the age of fifty who wish to enjoy later life to the fullest possibility. It is well written, clearly stated, and precisely on point relating to improvement and preservation of health, activity, and well-being.

The authors of *Active Aging*—Dr. Barbara McCool and Dr. Montague Brown—are my neighbors in the independent living section of a retirement facility named Bishop Spencer Place. We frequently go to dinner together, and we participate in other activities in the programming here, including exercise classes, musical programs, lectures on interesting scholarly subjects, and current events of our Greater Kansas City community and the nation. In the space of about four years, we have become close friends and shared ideas on many subjects, including religious beliefs, governmental issues, and, yes, political thought. We've also discussed ideas about active participation in life in later years, and I can vouch for the fact that they practice what they recommend.

The authors are an amazing couple. They've both studied extensively in postgraduate work and have applied in so many ways what they've learned. Over some time, each of them has earned four degrees from prestigious universities, which have prepared them for their teaching and leadership careers. The details of their higher education achievement can be found elsewhere in this publication.

Equally important is their extensive experience in teaching—as professors on related subjects, and lecturing and consulting extensively concerning health care issues. Their expertise is identified in later pages of this book.

The authors formed their own consulting firm and have appeared for many years as lecturers, discussion leaders, and advisors concerning health care issues and managing health care.

Throughout my personal life, I recognized, having been tutored by knowledgeable parents, the importance of exercise and sensible diet as both pertain to one's health. During my childhood and high school years, I probably ate everything I could get my hands on but was also participating in strenuous exercise in training and participation in athletic endeavors and summer work on my grandparents' farm. I served in the US Army in WWII and probably ate as much as I could of whatever was available but "wore it off" by performing assignments as required. After college, I continued the rather modest and irregular exercise of swimming, jogging, golf, and, of course, lots of yard work. These things seemed to keep me in relatively good health. However, I did not study or pay much attention to diet in the way outlined by the authors.

I wish now that during the middle and latter part of my life I would have had the benefit of the wisdom set forth in *Active Aging*. This book is really common sense, founded on the basis of moderation in all things but buttressed by intelligent analysis and evaluation by the authors, who have taken into account new discoveries, reports, procedures, and methods of extending productive life. They certainly have had the background and experience to make such recommendations.

I was privileged to read drafts of the written materials and make observations while the book was being formulated. The authors have worked hard and diligently to produce a very practical, understandable and helpful guide to aid and encourage the aging population to enjoy their later years to the fullest.

I am now officially old and somewhat impaired with a bad right ankle and foot, causing me to use a cane. However, I still go to my law office to do some work there three days a week, and I am active with several organizations, including my church choir. I also regularly exercise using appropriate machines in our facility, take vitamins, and enjoy an occasional Scotch.

My own parents lived to be quite elderly, so the adage about choosing your parents wisely is certainly pertinent. I have just recently celebrated my ninety-third birthday and am having a very good run. And now with the aid of *Active Aging* and the information therein, plus the support and supervision of the authors, I am shooting for at least another five years, and, with a bit of luck, maybe even beyond.

W. H. "Bert" Bates, BA, JD, JD HC
Resident at Bishop Spencer Place
Retired Lawyer with Lathrop Gage

CHAPTER ONE

Aging Is Mandatory. Acting Old Is Not.

Therein lies a tale
Shall we act our age stereotype?
What is best? Your reality, now!

Our dreams made manifest?
Hard to do? Do it anyway!!
Surely if we but grow and die
We can live fully until we die

*What you **WILL**, will be*
You can choose, you know
Choose to get stronger
Work to stay fit and lean
Dance, sing, pray, hope

Come friends
A glass of wine
Some drumming
Lean in, share our tale
Now is real
Embrace reality
Pay attention
Be kind, serve others

Introduction

In June of 2016, the question for us was, *What next?* Our cardiac rehabilitation exercise program had ended, and Monty had officially recovered; the brain fog from his 2015 cardiac bypass surgery was gone. And Barbara was recovering from her ordeal of managing our move from Tucson to Kansas City. In short, we were both recovering. The advice from the Cardiac Rehabilitation (CR) Team was, "Keep your exercise program going." We did that, in part, by continuing to use the CR Team's program (Barbara had begun a new exercise regimen for herself while supporting Monty) and beginning to take exercise classes at Bishop Spencer Place.

At our ages—then eighty-five and eighty-three—we were in the "Old Old" cohort. One of our most significant risk factors was, and still is, dementia. We thought one of the things that might best help to ward off that disease would be to keep our minds active. We needed a mental challenge, not merely a vacation or a casual course or two but a robust professional problem to solve. So, we decided to write a book on active aging, a long-delayed project that we'd often discussed but never begun in earnest.

We did not intend to write this book merely as a reflection of the past. We had an active life in Tucson and decided, "Let's do it in real time; let's task ourselves with the challenge of redesigning our lives for the older years." To do that would require challenging our mental capacity and stretching our cognitive resources and our ability to do the work for the book. It would be just what we needed to ward off decline and dementia. So we began.

The best is yet to come! If you don't believe this, you may be reading the wrong book. Now, as we approach eighty-six and eighty-eight, that is still our belief. Does this mean that things are more natural at an advanced age? Advanced age doesn't make things easier but age per se should not be a limiting factor for intellectual endeavors. We both obtained advanced degree after age 50. So why not write a book near 90? The problems of aging are more likely ones requiring daily attention, with the payoff being a higher level of good health rather than a new career or professional opportunity. The research and writing task is a lot of hard work, but as we edited the final product it is FUN! Even the editors admonition to do this or that, is interesting and a pleasure to be so engaged. If life span allows, perhaps there will be another book after age 90.

None of our chronic health conditions slow us down much, and we are still open to exploring new things in life. The calendar years are not what count the most. Our choices largely control our lives. We get to choose, and we choose to live actively while alive. Today, for example, we will sign up for a trip to begin ten months from now. By doing this, we affirm our intent to live fully, no matter our age or condition.

We have met people in their fifties and sixties who acted as if they were one step away from the nursing home. We also know people in their eighties and nineties who face life with a spring in their step and joy on their face. What makes the difference? Not their circumstances but how they respond to and shape life's events. A friend and mentor once told Monty, "If there is an elevator, take it; if a ride is offered for only a block or two, take it." That friend—a smoker—died at sixty-one of a heart attack. Can we say with any certainty that his failure to be more active in addition to smoking caused his early death? No, but our research does point to these factors as significant causes of heart disease. Not with certainty, but it provides us with an educated guess. Educated guesses are the best we can do.

Would simple measures such as walking and getting more fiber in the diet improve health? We think it is likely but not guaranteed. A positive attitude toward prevention and healthy living helps. Healthy aging demands acquiring knowledge and then applying that knowledge to every aspect of life—physical, mental, psychological, spiritual, and social. This book provides our assessment of such knowledge. We are not experts on the aging process, and, in fact, there may not be anyone who can offer comprehensive advice on the subject. However, we are lifelong learners who have dedicated ourselves to making the most of life, no matter how short or long it is. More importantly, we have lived using the ideas and methods discussed in this book. We have made our share of mistakes, corrected course, and moved on. In our question and answer sections for each chapter we will share our favorite sources for the material covered.

What This Book Is

- The personal journey of two people on a voyage of discovery.
- A review of insights from research.
- A wake-up call that it's never too late to engage in active aging.

What This Book Is Not

- A one-size-fits-all approach. Each of us—and each of you—must tailor a program that takes us from where we are to where we want to go.
- A motivational book. As much as we encourage you to engage in life, you will succeed only to the degree that you are self-motivated.
- The final word on active aging. Such a thing may never be written, since discoveries are being made and new chapters are being added daily.

The phrase "active aging" may sound trite to anyone experiencing the myriad challenges of growing old. We understand that it is tempting to let life pass on while we sit content to reflect on the early days. However, we refuse to go there, and so can you. Advancing age is a universal experience, and death is inescapable. We don't expect to live forever. We wrote this book because we wanted our years of living to be as healthy as possible. We are also of the opinion that we are more likely to be sure of what we think once we have written about it and have had it reviewed by others. Alternatively, as some might say, we aren't sure what we know until we have written it out and thought about it for a while.

Active aging brings great personal benefits by improving the quality of life. It keeps us engaged, and probably much longer than we would be otherwise. Also, we are less likely to need assistance from the limited individual, family, and public resources that provide care for the frail elderly.

Why Do We Need Active Aging? Consider the Numbers

The math for maintaining health and staying active is compelling. Caring for someone at home costs hundreds of dollars per day. Caring for them through assisted living costs $6,000 or more each month.

The income of average seniors living mostly on social security benefits is wiped out by any of these costs, which then pushes them onto Medicaid or other public support programs. The expense incurred for disability is high, but the loss of mobility that results from the inability to function is catastrophic for the individual and often for other family members as well. We are not immune to these forces; we could become bankrupt as well. In dollar terms, if one of us needed to be in assisted living or needed near full-time care, the cost would be more than double our current monthly fee.

Now consider that people are living longer than ever. Scientific advances have cut mortality for diseases that historically have had high death rates. And innovative organizational arrangements, such as Continuing Care Retirement Communities (CCRCs), allow seniors to seek other levels of care as they age.

With the baby boomer generation swelling the ranks of retirees at the rate of ten thousand a day, Medicare recipients create serious funding issues for governmental bodies.[1] With one-half or more of boomers having underfunded their pension savings, the impact on Medicaid costs will be severe.

Of significant concern for many families, aging people put a strain on the pocketbooks and calendars of their loved ones. Family members will find themselves heavily burdened, and many will need to take time away from jobs to provide care for elderly parents. For one of our neighbors, a daughter gave up a full-time job to help take care of her mother. The loss of that income is a burden. The time away from caring for her primary family is a burden. The price paid by the insurance system may well be less than the real cost to families for chronic disabilities. No rational person with less than many, many millions in savings can ignore the potential for financial collapse with potentially devastating life illnesses.

Such cost strains public financing and burdens boomer families. Health care services and facilities can be helpful, but the impact of these changes on lifestyle and disability from loss of function can be substantial.

Life extension continues apace. Living into the extremes of old age is no longer rare, and for some—like us—having successive careers, taking multiple "retooling" breaks, and continuing to find pleasure in work issues of lifelong interest is a reality. The choice for more people today to have various careers over the course of their lives may well become the necessity as life spans lengthen. Just as importantly, the experience is more exciting and enjoyable for those who meet the challenges of mastering the issues discussed here. Public facilities accommodate our friends in wheelchairs who can get to more events, but it isn't easy for the individual nor for others who must assist.

---

1 The primary source for this information can be found at https://www.ssa.gov

Early Steps to a Life Design for Active Aging in Our Eighties

It should be no surprise that our first concern is walking upright, moving independently, and being strong enough for travel! Can choice improve fitness and wellness at any age? The answer for nearly everyone is a resounding yes. As every physical therapist knows, with motivation and much work, even the most impaired person often can improve.

The average person spends years growing up, obtaining the necessary skills to be successful in the workplace, raising a family, working decades in a profession or industrial setting, and finally reaching the point in life where the children are gone. Those who were in their twenties when they had children and become empty nesters at fifty face ten to twenty-five years more of active work before retirement. For a parent who has taken time out to raise children, this might mean starting or restarting a career and having twenty to thirty years to master its challenges. For someone who has had twenty-five to thirty-five years in a job, it might mean retooling and beginning a second career or independent business for a few decades before retiring closer to eighty than sixty-two.

Here at our retirement center, a lawyer, a businessman, and a scientist go to work daily. A few others continue to do consulting and other business activities. Many who had no paid careers continue their philanthropic and civic duties long after age eighty. Often a volunteer does work related to their previous jobs; others assist people around them who need help.

Whatever your career and life trajectory, it is essential to ask:

- Should I commit to this phase in my life by taking charge and making plans for active aging?
- As I age, will I be in charge of my daily affairs to maximize the likelihood that my elder years evolve creatively?

> **Active aging means embracing all of life with a commitment to high-level wellness in the physical, intellectual, spiritual, emotional, professional, social, and environmental realms. Active aging is the antithesis of "I don't know how" or "I don't have . . . time, energy, money, or, I can't make friends."**

We've made our choice: it is to stay active. We are committed to living each day fully—cherishing each day, being grateful for each day. We do not intend to waste time waiting around to die. That is our current choice. An alternative might have been to take an extended vacation and settle into a leisure regimen. However, we did not choose that. We chose Active, and to us that means not only being careful about our health but also continuing to work on projects of our own and offering assistance where we can to others whose projects can utilize our talents in meaningful ways.

Do we have what it takes? Active aging requires a can-do attitude. Our research and experience show that improvement is possible for almost everyone if they are willing to work at making things happen. First, believe this, or, if you don't yet trust this, fake it until you can. Failure to act is a decision. Interestingly, those who are most active are also the ones with sufficient energy and creativity to volunteer to help others when needed. If you're going to be active, stay active at work or through volunteering; help others. We continue to find ways to help others and volunteer when aid is requested.

Our Journey
Did all of this begin in our eighties? No. The sense of our life planning and the journey began in earnest in our early fifties. In 1981, Monty

finished law school, and Barbara left a government job. For family reasons, we settled in Kansas City, Missouri, to establish and work out a new career. In this process, we used our skills and training to consult with hospital administrators and to speak publicly about topics within our expertise. Speaking grew into a consulting business, which continued until our first retirement in 1995. We didn't initially plan to work independently as consultants or to work in a partnership business. Our careers had been on separate tracks before this point. We made a life decision to live in Kansas City so Barbara could care for her mother as she, now alone, lived out her last years. Teaming in a consulting business grew out of the circumstances of our careers at that juncture. Life happens, and people cope.

Barbara's work in government and Monty's law school time were draining. Both of us felt the need to re-imagine our careers. From a business and work perspective, each of us had substantial expertise in designing health care systems, especially their strategic vision. In personal health, we are public health educated; thus, we always seek ways to promote wellness and disease prevention. So looking for ways to stay fit and live vibrantly became an active interest and issue for us. Our health care organizational expertise made independent consulting a natural career path to follow.

Also, it was necessary to be fit when making presentations to clients and the public. Much of a consultant's life is on stage, so being active and alert is a job requirement. Our first consulting assignments were mostly educational in nature and took full advantage of our experiences to date. More in-depth consulting and study projects came as we became better known as consultants rather than as academics.

Early in our Kansas City time, we attended a wellness program of St. Luke's Hospital. This program was our first formal introduction to wellness programs. The fact that a cardiologist and psychiatrist teamed to conduct it left a lasting impression of the connectedness of a healthy body and healthy brain and how the two influence each other.

We then read about and developed our opportunities for fitness. However, our work kept us traveling, missing proper nutrition, and finding comfort in food rather than exercise. Our growing consulting practice kept us on the road throughout the country, with each of us working in different cities other than at home during many days of most weeks. Our reading about aging was not our consistent practice. Over time, however, it did take hold and dramatically influenced our retirement years, including leading to this attempt to re-cast our lives to better conform to an active aging model.

When Barbara's mother died, we decided to move to Washington, DC, to be closer to the debates and policy action on health care. Kansas City is a lovely place to live but hardly in the mainstream of public health policy. Nor was it a crossroad of movement of potential clients for our business. In the process, we reduced our staff, kept small offices with a law firm, and worked mostly from our apartment in DC. With much of our work on the road and by doing the writing ourselves, we dispensed with secretarial and other staff and became independent professionals working from our home. No doubt, this move lead to a sense that we could depend more on our own efforts to stay healthy. For about ten years of our consulting practice, we used a lot of staff help, and the last few years we used almost none. However, not having a team meant more work for the two of use, which could lead to burnout with an attendant failure of our fitness efforts. We did face burnout, and our fitness suffered.

Our business model was that of solo practitioners. We always had a few clients. With most clients, we worked as a team. We tailored our designs for each client; we had no canned models or analytical products that could be applied directly to others. Just focusing on one client's needs at a time was a satisfying way to work, but it did little to build standardized models that we could later sell as an ongoing business. So we did not create a business; rather, we created a scholarly life sufficient for support but led mostly by our intellectual interest and not as a pathway to wealth but adequate for a good life and retirement.

Our time in Washington was limited. One big project that we took on in South Carolina necessitated much travel. That project lasted over a year, and it drained our already flagging energy; we needed a break. We were past age sixty and actively thinking about where to live in retirement once relieved of the burdens of working to earn a living. Staying active was a big part of that planning. We needed to reinvent ourselves for a new kind of living, so we ramped up our search for the next stage of our lives—a place to retire.

Neither of us expected full retirement at sixty-two, so we thought about some lesser alternatives to full-time work as consultants. Barbara wanted to explore hospice nursing, and I thought teaching might be work that would keep us active.

Taking the Plunge

Long before we planned to retire, we created a core framework for how best to live a healthy life and stay as fit as possible. Our criterion for a retirement location embodied this framework. Our education pointed to the real possibility that many aspects of personal well-being and life style are key to supporting an active, healthy life. Our consulting experience with many health care systems reinforced our academically formed views. Despite the setbacks in our ongoing wellness efforts, we continued to believe in the necessity of those efforts for us to realize a vibrant lifestyle after retirement.

Our consulting put us in direct contact with many chief executive officers heading their organizations. Over time, we observed how they spent their early retirement years. Some clung tightly to their workplace, often having an office and secretarial help. Their minor chores were often to help with fundraising. Others moved to golf locations and hit the links, regularly meeting up with other retired executives. Many could be seen walking or frequenting a gym, often daily. Most actually spent a fair amount of time exercising while still working at their jobs. Those who stayed active seemed the most satisfied with their lives, whether it was staying in the community where they headed a prestigious institution or whether they retired to a golfing community and stayed active there. Staying active was the key to a happier lifestyle.

Fortunately for us, work and education are at the core of our interests in learning and expanding our horizons. We are lifelong learners, which is an active process. Life is a journey, not a destination. For us, it was and continues to be a learning and growing journey that requires much physical activity along the way.

While consulting out of Kansas City, we engaged in a pro bono project in Florida to help a colleague. At the time, he was CEO of a prestigious hospital system, but he was on the verge of retirement. In his retirement, he took on a minor role in helping the organization he had once headed; his project was to interest the University of Florida and the Mayo Clinic in focusing on issues of aging. This work led to the establishment of a Foundation on Active Aging with a mission of generating support for work with seniors to encourage active aging.

Medical interests focus on diseases and services for the elderly but not on keeping them more active with physical, mental, social, and spiritual functioning while aging. This narrow focus seems to have created a gap that needs attention. So this gap became our focus for more writing and research and for how we lived our lives as we contemplated aging from our then mid-fifties working lives. Our work on active aging was mostly on a pro bono basis, rarely with any financial assistance for travel and time.

It is not surprising that medical institutions do not focus on wellness. Most people seek doctors and hospitals when they become very sick. In short, they first lose their healthy state and need help for repair and getting life back together. However, it is often too late for that to happen. Besides, just what one might prescribe for wellness and activity isn't always well known or agreed upon by various health professionals.

When the round of health care reform happened in 1993, much testing was considered mandatory for all insurance policies. These tests were labeled wellness measures, but they were mostly testing to detect diseases. Wellness, if it comes, will be a result of individuals keeping their bodies active and eating foods that contain the nutrients our cells require to function healthily. We think the ideal foods will be whole plant foods—mainly greens, veggies, fruits, grains, seeds, and nuts. To thrive, the individual must act to get essential exercise and nutritious meals. Perfection in exactly what to do, as well as when and how, in order to achieve wellness remains to be discovered. And yet, each of us should pursue the knowledge and resources to achieve wellness as a major life goal.

In short, there is no easily defined product or service called "wellness." For wellness to happen, it is up to the individual to get the best information they can find and craft a lifestyle to stay healthy.

What Is Active Aging?

Active aging is generally considered to be the process of optimizing opportunities for health, participation, and security to enhance the quality of life as people age. It applies to both individuals and population groups. Governments and nongovernmental organizations tend to look at overall populations' health, but our working definition of active aging brings the ideal down to the level of each person.

Active aging is a daily process of choosing to optimize opportunities for improving one's health and quality of life

For individuals, this means making lifestyle choices that enhance the likelihood that they will be healthy and self-sufficient. Much of the physical and mental differences between those who age more successfully and those who do not are due to lifestyle. Who doesn't want the following conditions in their life?

- Stable physical and mental functioning
- Low risk for disease
- Active engagement in life

Everyone is a candidate for this kind of life, and much of it results from the choices that we each make in how we lives our lives.

The idea is to be fit for a better daily life, and likely for longer than one might otherwise expect to live. The idea is to live that way until the end of life. Getting there requires managing one's life in ways that contribute to achieving the desired outcomes. Almost everything one needs for an active life is within an individual's capacity to exert significant control over. Much of health and wellness does not come about through what health care professionals, drugs, and procedures can provide for us. Many health and wellness factors are free, such as walking for exercise, water for drinking, sunshine, and more. Today, libraries and the internet are also available for research to everyone.

It is difficult, however, to separate fact from fiction. For instance, it is a manufactured fiction that humans need three meals per day plus snacks. One or two meals a day and no snacks might be healthier, but one doesn't read this often. In fact, it's hard to find any place, although there are hints of it in technical papers. Fasting is also showing up now in the medical literature and has been a recommended behavior of many religions. In primitive cultures, one meal a day might be the norm. However, in our North American society, more and more and more seems to be the norm, if one takes advertising as a beacon of truth. So yes, it is difficult to get useful information on diet and exercise.

Although others can do things to help us manage problems, much is under our control. We are concerned about the general health of the population, but, in reality, we mainly can offer help for ourselves and those who seek to use the knowledge and tools presented here. Finding what will work for individuals is a personal task that no one but each respective individual can do. We must each experiment to find the right balance just for us. Our journey and choices might work for you, but they are offered mainly to acquaint you with ideas for trying, not as prescriptions for use by everyone.

While much of life is under one's control, our individual genetic and epigenetic environments vary. Many individuals carry the burden of dealing with severe issues. Not everything can be brought under control by willpower and hard work. We each must deal with what we have. For those our age, it is easy to see a wide range of abilities and the struggle it is for those with varying degrees of abilities. However it is a joy to see that for even those most handicapped by extant conditions, there is still sufficient agency in their lives to compel them to exercise and do what they still can for themselves.

We are not all blessed with ample resources to have the broadest range of choices in how we carry out an active life. Many variables impact health. The level of one's education ranks at the top of the list of positive influences on functional health. We are both blessed with more than a customary amount of educational opportunity and skill development, which gives us distinct advantages. However, even those with a high school education or less can do all of the things we do to stay fit. We can travel longer distances and more often perhaps, but our curiosity and engagement in positive thought and work do not require financial means to accomplish. It is true, however, that resources saved for retirement years can make a massive difference in the range and quality of things available for maintaining an active life.

Tools for Designing an Active Life

Our work experience provided us with an extensive knowledge base for designing an active life, but the essential elements are open to everyone: We are what we eat, so nutrition is an area where individual choices are a significant factor. And physical fitness and mental fitness also are primarily within personal control.

> **One's personal choices and decisions are critical factors in maintaining health and well-being. Our bodies are naturally self-healing, and our lifestyles are the means for optimizing wellness and recovery from illnesses.**

We focus on positive things we must do for ourselves to stay well, get stronger, and live better. We've done little research on specific diseases; instead, our concentration has been on fitness, nutrition, diabetes, and dementia. We did read about particular illnesses and disability where vulnerabilities exist due to genetics or family history, and have studied the things one might use to avoid or slow the progression of such diseases; that is, we've attempted to prevent problems, not wait for them to occur. But we are more interested in the positive side of mental functioning, intellectual growth, and development—that is, brain fitness.

We are creative dreamers, authors, and educators, and the life of the mind is our life's work. Because of this, our professions and intellectual interest have probably helped us prevent or mitigate dementia to this point. Mental fitness is a focus in our lives and livelihood; it is of great concern for us and others in their later years of experience.

As part of mental fitness, the psychology of creativity and mood holds special interest for us. In our assessment, brain or mental fitness correlates positively with physical fitness. As more is learned about the importance of how our biome interacts with our brains, it seems obvious that we need to consider the interconnections among our various organs and systems. We are wholistic beings, and no doubt more than the sum of our parts. Although we don't know precisely how these things work, we share our own experiences for others to judge. What we offer are observations from the field of practice from two observers who continue to ask: What is happening here? What is the best course of action given these circumstances?

Pursuing the Goal

The goal of fitness in body, mind, and spirit leads us to highlight things that seem most relevant to our personal mission to live an active life. By following our learnings, we seek to be active until we die. But for what purpose?

Because this goal of active aging is shared by many, our story is about helping us and others achieve it. In general, if what we know and practice is correct, it will mean higher energy, mobility, and sense of well-being—physically, socially, psychologically, intellectually, and spiritually throughout life.

There is a big caveat attached to the sharing of our story: each person is different. Life is an experiment with a study population of N=1! Also, the science of what is best is often incomplete and rarely based on the kind of studies needed to prove causation. At best, much of the science is based on speculation about causation inferred from correlational studies. Our case study is the same. It is only our story. It may provide ideas anyone may try, but it isn't proof of anything except that, to the extent our memories are intact, it happened to us.

However, life isn't just about living well, and it isn't just about living longer. **LIFE is about an overarching purpose.** It is about keeping our energy up to continue our work. Each of us has things we feel are worth living for and accomplishing, such as raising a family, painting a great picture, providing for our loved ones, building an organization, or being a compassionate person. For others, life's purpose might be less about a particular object and more about abstract ideals, such as living an ethical and religious life.

To have a purpose in life means to have some overarching sense that life is meaningful and to be lived or used toward some higher end. Our work in health care, for instance, carries with it a sense that what we are doing will advance the cause of better health for people. In a more precise manner, the jobs we did always had that element of developing the purpose of improving health for all. For Barbara, who provided direct care to patients, this maxim has been self-evident. In retirement, she went back to serving hospice patients. For Monty, the first post-retirement work was a teaching assignment for health administrators. Early on, these professional purposes were at the core of our efforts.

We both found these jobs too fatiguing, however, and fell back on our long-term interest of active aging. If we were to help others, our own health had to be good. "Active" did not at this stage mean more of the same but more attention to our health since one who becomes infirm is less able to help others. Our focus shifted more to improving our fitness and well-being. At a minimum, we had to be well enough to care for one another. That seems as much the case today as it did early in our retirement.

Active aging is a commitment to continually strive for positive well-being as we seek physical, intellectual, psychological, and spiritual wellness. We do this for its own sake as well as for keeping us fit to fulfill our higher purpose. It is a stance toward life that encompasses feeling alert and energizes us daily. It requires that we stay mindful of our body, mind, and spirit in the context of our environment and the people with whom we interact. While seeking a high level of wellness, we do not expect to return to some golden age of fitness and high energy. Still, in doing this for ourselves, we do it for all people.

"Wellness" is another commonly used term referring to health in body, mind, and spirit. It is associated with the idea of intentionally doing things to prevent illness and achieve a better quality of life with fewer years of disease or disability, or perhaps even a few more years of life. Wellness is associated with the idea of preventing illness and disability through conscious efforts. Active aging is a pursuit of wellness through living an active lifestyle.

Our several approaches to finding more professional work were moderately successful, but we both knew that without personal renewal, these efforts would be less than our best performances. Instead of pushing on with work, we went in another direction that would take into account our lagging health and vitality.

We decided to work on fitness and doing the things in our desert home that would enhance our daily living and restore our sense of well-being and health. While we had kept up generally with scientific progress regarding achieving and maintaining an active lifestyle, we began reading even more and picking out projects to make our lifestyle more healthy and vibrant. We hiked, joined a Tai Chi class, took some spinning classes, and did yoga. We also became involved in our local community. In short, we implemented a progressive aging agenda.

Active Aging Agenda

Active aging includes these essential dimensions:

- **Physical:** strength, flexibility, endurance, balance, exercise, habits, and diet
- **Psychological**: purpose, motivation, self-esteem, and mindfulness

- **Intellectual**: mindfulness, creative thinking, modeling, feelings, consciousness, and success strategies
- **Social/community**: building connections and keeping them active
- **Spiritual**: purpose in life, meditation, serving others, and relationship with a Higher Being

Throughout this book, we present ideas and methods for solving some of the problems we faced in our aging journey. We discuss the frameworks, problem-solving, and tools we used for some of the real issues we had to deal with in our own mission.

Our environment has varied according to our educational choices, school, work life, family obligations, social engagements, and retirement choices. Our constant challenge is to find ways to correlate our life plan for where we live and the services we might need for ourselves and for serving others. The tools and means vary, and many are abundantly available in our society.

On most days we grapple with issues of what to eat, exercises to do, how to engage socially with others, what of our creative pursuits will get done. In addition there are ongoing issues of community, family, faith and activities of daily living to consider. In all of these pursuits the issues of active aging are involved. We have many ways of thinking about the mind/body/spirit beings that we are. But life is far more complicated than we often imagine, and we cannot reduce it to a few elements. Humbling as that is to say, it only expresses our profound amazement at the unique creatures that we imagine ourselves to be. Staying vibrant for the expression of our lives is fundamental to carrying out whatever purpose we have chosen (or had chosen for us) in life.

A Means, Not an End

We discuss things needed for particular forms of movement, thought, or activity. Much that we write about are means, not ends in themselves, which is a more abstract approach to life. For instance, exercising the body creates conditions for changes in the brain, and those changes likely relate to circumstances that decrease the elements associated with dementia. Some things are done because of very real concerns for maintaining one's balance. If we are to travel in the future, our strength needs to be maintained at a high level, sufficient to put the 30 pound bag in an overhead bin.

Fitness can also improve self-esteem, which, in turn, can have positive effects on social relations. We exercise to be able to pursue life's purpose and its critical goals, and this leads us to a better quality of life. These chains of connection require some overlap in exposition. They also make a more significant point: exercise is an essential lifelong habit necessary to improve the quality of our lives. Fitness is closer to that which people have sought over the ages—the secret to living, not forever but better and longer.

Finally, this book is part of our journey to more fully grasp and record what it means to age actively. As we research it, live it, and model it, we are questers. The story told here is our best estimate of what is required to age actively. By writing it all down and sharing it with others, we are inviting others to use what we're sharing, to critique it with us, and to improve their lives and ours. It is a collaboration to be shared and developed. One of life's central purposes is to share one's journey. This book serves that purpose.

CHAPTER ONE (Q&A)

1. Why should anyone care about Active Aging?

Do you want a life free from disease and decrepitude, or one which is filled with lots of vitality, good energy, and independence of movement, thought, and companionship? Staying active is the way to achieve excellent health and wellness essential to an independent existence and the ability to help others when needed.

We have known this throughout our professional careers. It is general knowledge, though we have lapsed often in doing all the things we recommend.

2. When should one begin preparing for Active Aging?

Now! In the present! TODAY! One of the most significant impediments to good health is inactivity. So move more, ache less; work more; work and play with greater ease. Movement is the key to life. We are aware that for any recommendation, there will be limits on how much one can do without injury and how little one can do to achieve no impact. Like everything else in life, all recommendations have limits; they are dose dependent. How much is just right for you is always a question to ask yourself.

What would be the easy way to begin this journey? Just do a bit more each hour, each day, each week. Walk instead of riding an elevator or riding in a car. If you spend much of the day sitting, get up and move around for ten minutes each hour. If you live in an apartment building, walk up and down a few floors or go outside and walk around the block a few times daily.

In our working years, we often did things to stay active and move more. Regular exercise came and went in our lives. We became more active in our forties, knowing that it was necessary for our health, although work situations made it difficult at times.

3. **Are there things beside movement and working out that are needed for Active Aging?**

Good, fresh food that is light on meats and fish, loaded with colorful vegetables, berries, nuts, and plenty of water is the best choice. Avoid extra sugar and salt, which are often found in an overabundance in manufactured foods. Monty cut sugar and bread from his diet, along with deserts. Fruit, with its fiber, is an excellent substitute for sweet desserts.

Was this easy on the road? NO! And many times we grab a burger, fries, and shake from a carry-out window—a potent stress reliever and opportunity to get home from work and crash.

4. **Is there more?**

Yes, a pleasant social life, purpose and spiritual peace, intellectual acuity, and more. And yes, get a good night's sleep. Our bodies— especially the brain—require the rest in order to process the events of the day, clear debris, and clarify those nagging questions. Many days after a good night's sleep, the puzzle of the day before presents an answer upon awakening. How much sleep is needed? Eight hours is often suggested, but the quality is also essential. We aim for eight hours at night and usually a nap in the afternoon.

During our dozen or more consulting years, we often slept in hotel beds, many of which were uncomfortable, and our hours off the job were too few to get proper rest. At home, we did better, but work requirements often conflicted with adequate sleep patterns.

In our retirement setting, better sleep is more tranquil, although when we lived in the desert with cats and dogs, the animals' lives often dictated our sleeping and waking hours. Fortunately, our animals loved naps as much as did we. So that also helped.

5. Are there other reasons to seek Active Aging?

More people are living with chronic diseases that stem in part from not actively aging and having far too little savings for their needs in later years. Being active can reduce the cost to individuals, families, and society of the burdens of taking care of frail, needy persons who, but for the earlier lack of self-care, might take care of themselves.

Also, in old age, spouses and other family members who are aging themselves find it necessary to give up income, work, and leisure to care for those who have needs beyond their capacity to care for themselves.

In short, everyone benefits when each of us takes a prudent course of good self-care by keeping fit and working harder to stay active and independent. And, yes, every time it is hard to recover. But taking it only one day at a time, with repetition each day, higher levels of functioning return. Nothing reverses things forever, so stay modest; just do the right things today, and that is sufficient.

6. Is Active Aging something everyone should be doing? Can everyone do it?

We assume that everyone wishes to live the best and healthiest life possible. So a resounding YES to the question of whether Active Aging is something everyone should be doing. And everyone has a baseline from which they can improve with effort and intention, although nature serves up individual differences that can be profound.

7. Will everyone do these things?

Sadly, it seems unlikely that everyone will engage in active aging. We have kept our practical aging efforts going well—but off and on! And that was in the face of years of education and working in the health fields where the knowledge of what to do is widespread. Many things militate against taking responsibility for one's own health, not the least of which are the products and services sold to make the job easier or recovery from problems easier. Everyone has the opportunity to do more for themselves. Our advice? Just do it. Don't obsess over the notion that it is for life; make today a more fabulous day by having a pleasant experience. Remember, life is just one day at a time. There are only memories of yesterdays and dreams of tomorrows. What is real is today.

8. You stress the importance of doing things in the present and acting on what is in front of you in that present moment. What are the reasons for this?

One reason is that people often get stuck repeating their experiences of past events or worrying about future events. If this stickiness happens too often, it may be referred to as depression or anxiety disorder. People tend to obsess about bad things that occurred in the past or about bad things that might happen in the future. By focusing on the present, both debilitating behaviors can be avoided.

9. Are there things not done that you might do differently if time were reversed?

Throughout this book, we stress not obsessing over the past because it cannot be changed. Still, the question of what we might have done different is a fair one. Yes, it would have been helpful to have done much earlier more of the things we now do. Exercising regularly is one. Eating more real foods, with less emphasis on animal protein is another. Having a deeper and more frequent mediation practice would have smoothed some parts of life. And doing this level of research into life design for health would have helped to spot the errors in science reporting, government guidelines, and human practices. Perhaps this book would be one of a series of volumes written every five years or so to deal with the twists and turns of science and policy.

10. You don't use a lot of footnote to show where the ideas covered may be found. Are there sources, you found most useful here?

Some ideas cut across many areas of past studies and some relate to cultural features of our families. Many features of our family lives stressed self reliance and doing things for oneself. For Monty work was an early feature of life, with jobs and income as early as age 8 or so. For Barbara the culture of religious orders in her schooling set examples of service and self reliance at an early age. For both, years of education led to insights on behaviors which aid people in achieving better lives. Education in public health focused more on health than curative medicine.

Both have benefitted from the work of Carl Rogers in psychology, Andrew Weil in Integrative Medicine, Mark Hyman, MD, Functional Medicine, Michael Greger M.D. nutritional sciences, and many, many more. All of these names can be found on search engines and YouTube videos of their ideas. Readers should look for them and try some of the subjects they cover. Singling out which one contributed to our understanding of the trends in the field is impossible for us to untangle.

11. It is common to provide citations for ideas and facts quoted from other sources, but few are found here. Would it not be helpful to do more of that here?

One of the facts that was given earlier was the generally reported fact baby boomers are retiring in great numbers. When that number was first read it was probably in all of the three papers we read daily, the NYTimes, Wall Street Journal and the Washington Post. That number came from a report out of the Social Security Administration. And their news release quoted a report to that agency. Instead of providing a specific citation, primary, secondary or tertiary we suggested using the Social Security Website to obtain more primary data on the general subject. We encourage broader reading and more research and do not intend our assimilated data and insights as primary sources except for our views on the subject. With such primary sources the reader going there and being more familiar with their offerings, we believe, is a better step to take than merely taking that one number as the essence of the issues it raises.

CHAPTER TWO

Staying Fit: Exercise Your Rights

Get Fit, stay Fit
Exercise Your Rights, chose to be fit
Get fit, stay fit relative to your abilities
Healthy is fit to work, play, serve
When to do it? NOW

Food is fuel for the body
Fresh is best
Bright colors, cooked the least
Tubers, fruit, greens, beans
Debates rage

Sugar, Salt, Fats,
Meat, fish, or plants only?
Life is a one-person experiment
Study the science, try the ideas most appealing
Pick ones that work for you
What shall we do?
Make a difference
Have a Purpose
Develop your talents
Share your gifts

Initial assumptions

In general, the human body begins in reasonably good working order. It is intact and ready to start life. It seeks nourishment supplied by the mother and begins its growth cycle. Also, it seems equipped to be self-adjusting and healing. If cut, it bleeds and healing begins without other interventions. With the development of medicine, and even before our modern arrays of therapies, there might be a mother who aids the repair and healing processes or a shaman or a physician. But at the core of our being, we are equipped with the necessary mechanisms for self-repair.

In Monty's early studies, he found professional recommendations to give the patient up to two weeks to self-repair. After a brief description of a problem, the answer would be something like this, "Take aspirin if pain persists, drink lots of water, and come into our office for an exam if the problem persists." Much of what is needed for the body to maintain itself is found by working the body, nourishing it with whole-plant foods, and being supported by loving family and friends. The individual can, in short, become captain of their own destiny by taking charge and doing those things that will help the body in its growth and self-repair mode. Exercising to stay fit is one of those must-do things.

Stay Fit

Determining when we are aging doesn't require much guesswork. Our bodies let us know. Neither of us played a significant sport. Our exercise was mainly walking from house to car and from parking lots to an office or to a store. When Monty finished law school, and Barbara left government work, we moved to Kansas City to begin the next stage of our professional careers. We were around fifty at that time. Without a pre-determined path to follow, we did an initial assessment. Among our most important goals was personal fitness. Our pensions also needed to be improved, and Barbara needed to stay close to care for her mother.

Upon arriving in Kansas City, we began consulting, following up on clients Monty had during his law school years. Consulting meant more travel and, thus, uneven fitness regimens and poor eating and sleeping habits—all of which are danger areas for older people who wish to avoid the diseases that stem in part from unfitness as they age.

We weren't ready to retire because we hadn't saved enough to afford retirement. Monty with his newly minted law degree was ready to work on new problems with a deeper and broader perspective than he had before. Barbara was ready to find a new career or try out her skills as a consultant.

So we began a new career outside of universities and, at the same time, began to seriously consider how to best live the next stage of life before retiring from active work. Like everyone else, we began to seriously consider our need for retirement financing, make adjustments, to be ready for the time when income becomes the social security check and the withdrawal of savings put aside for later years. That was a minimum. Questions, questions . . . where to live, what to do, how to ensure and maintain health, and when health goes, what next? Life is more about questions than answers. Also, it is more about the process than the final answers.

We believed that we needed to have health insurance and that being self-employed would make that an issue for us. We needed a plan to stay healthy. We also knew that being healthy was our responsibility, not something we could not buy from others nor find in ordinary medical practices. In Kansas City, we explored possibilities with colleagues and participated in a fitness program run by a local hospital. The plan had trainers and all kinds of equipment and fitness classes. Monty got into a class, and his trainer advised doing more walking. Shortly after he began that exercise routine, he suffered a stress fracture injury while walking at a public park near our home.

The cause of that fracture was not only the walking but also walking while obese! The orthopedic surgeon said, "We don't see this type of injury often except with young soldiers who are carrying eighty pounds of gear on their backs." Whereas the soldier's excess weight was in his backpack, Monty's excess pounds were inside his body. So doing the right thing can also become a liability. That fractured femur did not end our working out, but it set us back a year or so.

We, like many people, have been in and out of phases of getting into shape and then recovering from times of relative stress and neglect of our physical well-being. Friends and relatives suffer the same cycles. A younger brother of Monty's had a bout with cancer caused by x-rays to treat acne. His brother, like Barbara's parents, was hypertensive. Such events touch many lives. Some of these ups and downs are avoidable and some not, but most can be anticipated and mitigated by learning about and using healthy behaviors. It is no accident that our retirement home was within walking distance from the Saguaro National Park (SNP). We often hiked in areas open for human use. Most of SNP is wilderness and closed to humans. When living in the area, we walked the roads adjacent to the park and hiked trails inside the SNP. Membership in a local YMCA, Tai Chi, and yoga enhanced those activities. Our own four-plus-acre lot offered many outdoor activities, including swimming.

By contrast, this plan for being out and in natural environments is entirely different from what will work as age and the increased likelihood of impairments and slowing down occurs. In the city we have no seashore or national park. Nor are the road rocky and unpaved. Here we have most of our fitness inside or at a fully service gym. We needed more protection, more training on correct methods for using equipment. In short we need to stay fit while doing so in a sheltered environment.

Now in our second retirement and living at Bishop Spencer Place, a Life Plan/Continuing Care Retirement Center (LP/CCRC), in Kansas City, Missouri, fitness is encouraged, with exercise classes and facilities convenient to our living quarters. During our working years and early retirement, fitness was the principal protector against the problems associated with aging. Age is associated with the many conditions listed on our medical charts. Active aging is the antidote to the many downsides to aging. Walking and eating fresh foods is at the core of our programs. Walking led to our significant engagements. It is also in community fitness programs that work for us. For others, their exercise comes through tennis, golf, swimming, and other such activities.

Apartment buildings offer stairs for the more fit, hallways for those who can't handle stairs, and elevators when walking become difficult. Classes and other local places are available for more. But nothing in the city matches the beauty of the great out-of-doors in natural settings.

Necessities, Not Choices

Fitness activities were never meant to be options, because humans are not designed for leisure and sedentary lifestyles. Would we have been better off doing more exercises before retiring? Of course, the answer is yes. But we also think it is never too late to begin. And, for those not yet so engaged, today is a good time to start.

> **We need strength, flexibility, stamina, and more. These are necessities, not choices.**

In short, "use it or lose it" isn't some theory of what will happen in the future. It is ever-present, never a real choice unless someone is ready to transition to canes or walkers and assistance with daily living.

Old age can be a blessing or a curse, depending heavily upon what people do to remain fit. If a significant setback occurs (heart surgery, for instance), as soon as conditions permit, begin the journey back to health. It may take months or even a year or more, but it is merely the journey of life. It must be done to live as fully and actively as possible after a setback.

Our Natural Condition

Long before we evolved into the human forms we know today, we were small clusters of cells, and before that, simple few-cell creatures. We developed as both self-feeding and self-healing or died off. Long after we evolved into a human form, we remained self-dependent for all our needs, including healing. We are virtually self-sufficient, or, at least, once were. Perhaps with agriculture, we began to see people specializing and living more in clusters, organizing around specialization and exchange among specialists for more and more of our needs, but our natural condition is self-sufficient and self-healing. Medical and other specialists can help, but our first line of good health comes from self-management and our natural healing systems.

Human animals moved to meet their daily needs. Hunter-gatherers made long treks, with sudden bursts of speed required for survival. No doubt many days were filled with digging and just gathering roots and berries. It should not be surprising that effective exercise regimens mimic this necessity, which is our genetic basis for life. Later, as humans became farmers, herdsmen, and child-bearers, hard daily work was the norm. In the modern era, much of the hard physical work of life is absent for most, which creates our need for substitutes for the more natural conditions now absent.

Today, work for many involves sitting, using the mind more than the body. We need to find ways to keep entire life systems going. Our bodies, our greatest human asset, absolutely require lots of activity, including bursts of activity that challenge our systems.

> **The key to modern living isn't to go back to ancestral ways but to find physical activities that we can pursue to keep the body/ mind in shape to thrive.**

We tend to forget that our body is a self-healing organism. To keep the body working well requires that we keep it moving, staying active or carving out time to exercise. In nature, things not used atrophy, fail, or fall away. Life is frugal, and holding on to things neglected or not used is wasteful. So we can't count on keeping strength or good brain power if we neglect to keep it in good working order. It is natural to forget that which you do not use. "Use it or lose it" is a powerful message often neglected. At our age, continuing to work means that we are more likely to work and ignore rest and recreation. Relaxation is healthy, and, in our past, we often neglected it.

Who Benefits from Fitness?

The question is not so much who benefits from improved fitness but who doesn't? Do what you love or can come to love and go from there. Work at it. Build on it. Become stronger, and stay that way longer. There are many ways to keep moving, so doing that which pleases you the most has the best chance of remaining important in life. Daily activities offer many ways to stay fit. Barbara walks to deliver minutes from meetings and to meet with committee members. Monty takes the stairs rather than the elevator. Could we do more? Yes, we should. We should also do more vacations and take more frequent forays into natural settings that provide fresh vistas for our minds.

Fitness is likely the most essential active-aging goal of all:

- Fitness for the brain
- Strengthening for the heart
- Fitness for weight control

- Uplifting for the spirit

From time to time, we need to repair one or more of our natural systems. We have experienced Barbara's knee and hip repairs, and for Monty, stress fracture of the femur and heart surgery. Each caused setbacks to fitness regimens, so each required recovery. Moreover, each would have been handled better had we been in better shape before the event happened. However, for all, it is necessary to balance the need of the body to self-repair with the need to continue striving to extend the ability to stay strong. We have seen no studies showing exercise as the cause of chronic diseases. Of course, one can incur injuries, and overdo even the best of things, so be careful and consult experts in areas as you embark on new regimens.

Exercise and fitness are essential for weight control, mental functioning, and alertness. Indeed, exercise and human fitness influence every subject in this book in one way or another. More precise advice for each of us on exactly what to do is best left to personal assessments by our caregivers and exercise professionals.

Keep in mind that pushing yourself to sweat, feel the burn or notice exertion is required. A slow, light stroll is a pleasure but fails the sufficiency test.[2] Find the right exercise for you. It should be fun and match your abilities. A friend who is recovering from a stroke, uses his walker to walk a few hallways daily. He also spends time on a Nustep machine and resistance bands for upper body toning. He is getting stronger, and his mood is positive and upbeat. No doubt his will to do this is and his movement is helping him get stronger. We do much of the same without the injury recovery as a motivator. This is merely what one at our age should do.

---

2   Gibala, Martin. (2017). The One Minute Workout. New York: Penguin Random House Group. Latest books strongly suggest High Intensity Interval Training for optimal use of time. We use it for our aerobic routines and often on walks..

Is Physical Fitness for You?

Physical Fitness can be a defining passion, a cherished sport, or simply an activity. It is cultivated, practiced, and considered an essential function each day to carry out the activities of daily living. Should we consider physical fitness as more or less critical than other passions and duties? More, it seems to us. Unless we maintain our functioning at a reasonably high level, it becomes impossible to do other things. Being out of shape when caretaking burdens overtake one's life makes it harder to aid another and much harder to get the time to stay fit. Get fit early, and try to keep healthy throughout your life.

At our retirement center, we exercise together, often in classes with others. We find that over time much of our socializing is with people who share in those group activities. Some can and do embark on exercise regimens alone and never go to class. Find what works for you. Socializing via exercise is a bonus for us.

Taking care of a spouse takes precedence over many other things and can become an essential duty. However, care-taking should not stop our fitness efforts. Unless we maintain our fitness level, we cannot be of much help to others. Assisting a loved one's exercise helps both.

Caregivers often resist taking care of themselves. Especially in light of this, it is wise to establish patterns of fitness that are well understood as essential to maintain before infirmity occurs. Plan for it, and discuss it as part of life planning. We all need activities and life projects that keep us motivated and in vital health. Did we do all of this well ourselves? No, but we wish that we had done so. By heeding this advice, we will be better prepared for the next time!

Physical fitness lays a solid foundation on which programs can build. You will be on the road to a more-active life, a life with more joy and more happiness, and you will be more of an inspiration for others as well.

It's easy to see and feel the benefits of physical fitness and thus feel confident in recommending it to others. Feeling good, thinking more clearly, enjoying the ability to walk at a good pace—all coming from a renewed and expanded view and commitment to fitness—is great. Most days for us are great days. Physical fitness is now a critical factor in managing the good life we lead on our aging journey.

Find Your Path

Everyone must find for themselves what they need and what priorities they must follow. Our approach may not fit everyone, so design your own approach or see one suggested by others.

Are you worried about dementia or clear thinking in your later years? Fitness likely is one great answer to these issues. Exercise can help repair many organs and functions. Brain function improvements, for one, can come from activity. It is no accident that most writers on the subject of wellness for aging adults mention caring for mind, body, and spirit to prevent, mitigate, or cure many of the problems we face.

This message of both encouragement and warning often is shared by fitness buffs. Muscle loss begins early in adulthood and keeps going down unless a person takes decisive steps to keep it from shrinking too far too fast. Many changes attributed to aging are caused in large part by lack of use. The loss of muscle mass slows, however, when one is active; we can mitigate age-related loss and maintain strength longer by using our muscles more.

"Use it or lose it" is true both in an individual lifetime as well as in a genetic evolutionary time. Watch the Senior Olympics sometime, and any sense that handicaps prevent fitness fade fast. Alternatively, watch the Paralympics and see how those who have significant losses perform.

Whatever your passion and whatever your duties, any ground lost to the ongoing deterioration of muscle from aging slows with exercise and proper diet. Doing the desired work for the heart or brain requires doing work for the whole body. It is possible to tweak one muscle group at a time to help that muscle, but the heart and significant organs benefit most when doing full body work such as jogging or swimming.[3] Doing what you can when you can is the best time to start. The sooner, the better, but there is no time beyond which one cannot begin or, after faltering, cannot begin again.

Monty remembers a study he read about when still doing research at the University of Chicago. It was conducted in a New England nursing home, and the subjects were all in their nineties. They used strength training, and all of the participants gained strength compared to a control group.[4] There seems to be no age limit to the ability of humans to build muscle with serious work.

There are many good ways to exercise, many of which we have tried. Our main exercise, however, is walking. Before our retirement in Tucson, we prioritized being close to nature to walk on rough ground, in the open air, and around other creatures. Unfortunately much of our work and hobbies are done in a sitting position.

Humans are designed to walk to carry out life activities. By adding a sprint or fast pace to a nature walk, one mimics the efforts of Paleolithic ancestors—walk to stalk, dash to kill. Today we call that kind of walk interval training. Our genes support a wide variety of speeds,

---

3   https://www.mayoclinic.org/why-interval-training-may-be...workout.../art-20342125
4   https://www.ncbi.nlm.nih.gov/pmc/articles/PMC6343518/

stops, and starts. Today's exercise programs can mimic quick changes in pace that nature often required of our ancestors.

We are now in our mid-eighties and living with many who are older. For all of us, the exercise of walking must be supplemented with squats and leg muscle exercises that will enable us to get in and out of chairs. Ankle and leg muscle weakness and balance problems cause falls, especially among slow walkers.

Variety Is the Spice

Recommendations vary regarding how much to exercise. Our preference is daily exercise with at least three days of it having substantial strength training, including upper body, lower body, and core exercises. Some days we do two forty-five-minute classes, some bike time for interval training, and walking.

We work on endurance, balance, strength, and flexibility. All are important. Walking, gardening, pushing a lawnmower or any strenuous movement can elevate your heart rate to improve heart, lung, and circulatory functions. By doing the hard work, the whole body (brain included) benefits. All movement helps because endurance requires a bit of a stretch, a push beyond your average pace. To get the most significant gain from walking, move briskly as though you need to be somewhere very soon! Barbara gets much exercise working a committee of volunteers that she directs. Monty does less walking but adds heavy-duty intervals to his machine workouts. Exert yourself. Get the sweat going, the heart rate up, and the breathing a bit labored.

Walking leads the list of exercises most readily available to everyone. It is an excellent endurance exercise. If you are doing just ten minutes at a time, do three or more sessions a day. Thirty minutes a day is considered sufficient. Overall, an hour a day is regarded as a better bet to achieve more significant weight loss, and six days a week with some hard work for half of that hour. We both get an hour a day, six days a week, or more. Climbing stairs in an apartment building and doing interval training when walking provides a good hour of work. Remember—a ten-minute break to exercise per hour to avoid the damage from too much idle time. In short, keep moving.

Maintaining or Rebuilding Muscle

Strength training also is essential. Lifting capacity, carrying groceries or travel bags on and off airplanes, and, at some point, getting up and out of chairs can become a test of strength. There are many ways to increase resilience. Weightlifting is the most obvious, and you don't need a gym to get started. Countertop pushups are an easy way to build some muscle groups. If you're in the bathroom or kitchen, do some squats at a counter. One of our favorites is doing sit-ups from a chair, which is a muscle challenge. Pick one or more such exercises, and get moving.

Muscles and tendons need stretching after warming up a bit. Our trainers recommend at least a day between muscle-building workouts. Every exercise uses some muscles. So for us, that extra day in between is reserved for heavier workouts on specific muscle groups. Feeling a stretch, being a little sore the next day, or minor pain sensations are considered evidence of growth, not injury. We never try to push into the pain zone. So we confess: we play it relatively safe on most things. Moderation is more of our approach.

Stay Balanced

Exercise also addresses balance. Poor gait and weak leg muscles are the main culprits in falls. Walking in your house on your toes for a bit and then on your heels for a bit is a great way to work some of your most critical balancing muscles. All strength training helps with balance, but Tai Chi is best known for improving balance and it's our main exercise for balance. Balance in life generally is essential. At retirement, if not before, exercise should become as routine as brushing one's teeth.

Exercise daily in some form, at least every other day for strength workouts.

Stretch Yourself

Stretching is a significant form of exercise that is critical for ease of movement, especially when the action is a bit awkward, unusual, or surprising. How many ankle sprains, rotator-cuff injuries, and other such injuries are the result of sudden unanticipated movement? Circumstances often require mobility and flexibility that isn't available when needed.

Stretching is essential for flexibility. Which muscles need it? Every muscle needs stretching. Our morning classes begin with warming-up movements, which are followed by strengthening routines and then stretching.

Fitness Is An Ideal For A Healthy Life

To build your personal exercise program, research, study, evaluate, make some choices, and begin with a strong desire to be fit. Select routines that build as you gain strength, endurance, and flexibility. Fitness should be on your agenda, even if you are not concerned about active aging. We got the message before our first retirement; now, in our second retirement, it remains a big priority albeit one with many differences from our outdoor life in the mountains, valleys, and deserts of Arizona.

Feeling fit is terrific at every age. However, being able to walk to dinner is considered a blessing at eighty-five-plus. We see neighbors who have pursued sports for years; they get up quickly, walk fast, take stairs, and help others as well. Others use small carts for transport to the dining areas and walking sticks to get to a table. It is often a matter of great pride to make that last effort to walk to a table. Many who try to walk to dinner are the same ones who exercise to keep moving. The sooner one takes fitness seriously, the better able they will be in older ages to walk to a table and sit in regular chairs rather than being confined to a mobile platform.

Fitness Barriers

Are there any excuses that we haven't tried? Is it too cold, windy, or hot outside to take a walk? After reading about alternatives, it is easy to select something to fit into the schedule.

While working at universities and in our first consulting practice offices, we drove to work from home. Little walking was required. In Washington, DC, we got lots of walking by using the subway, which offered walking and stair climbing as well. In Tucson, we walked outside and took classes in Spinning, Tai Chi, and yoga. We both progressed significantly for about a year. Our instructors left, however, and we did not pursue other courses.

But failing to go once, twice, or more times is no excuse for never trying again. As one wag put it, "Fake it until you make it." Do it until it becomes a regular habit. Do it for yourself, do it for your loved one, do it because it is the right thing to do. We have begun again with Tai Chi classes and find it a good friend and most helpful exercise. Spinning has given way to treadmills, Nustep, and elliptical machines. All of these devices enable us to stay more fit for our aging journey.

Like many people, we almost always had fitness in our New Year's resolutions, and, also like many, we quit working out routinely after a few weeks. Life planning needs more than general goals and annual recommitments to those goals.

We realize that life-changing goals such as weight loss and exercise are the kinds of goals and commitments that must be renewed daily. Bite-size, not grandiose, wins the day. The tortoise verses hare race is won one step, one day at a time.

If you fail on any given day, forgive yourself, and don't do it two days in a row. We must begin again and do it one day at a time. There is always the temptation to say, "Let's take a short vacation and discuss this again." Avoid that temptation. Of course, a decent list of ways to fail could be much longer. Suffice it to say; we have failed often. However, we are still returning for another effort. Now living in retirement, we have the time, opportunity, and urgent necessity to get things right. There will be time enough to be dependent on caregivers. We cherish our independence.

New Beginnings

Fitness routines often are interrupted. Setbacks are fairly common, and some injuries, while not inevitable, are not unusual. Both underscore another major fact:

There will be setbacks and the need to begin again.As the old saying goes, if at first you don't succeed, try, try again. That wisdom advice applies after many new beginnings and many failures.

Although injury often results in caution, beginning again is a must-do behavior because stopping would mean staying on the treadmill of slow but steady decline. Life is a process, and the goal is to work daily to build and maintain a fit body and a bright, working mind. Each setback requires new thinking about what to do and how to do it, and building a step-by-step refreshed set of routines. That is an essential goal, every time. Just as our mistakes are often our best teachers, our injuries teach what we must avoid. Working out correctly to improve performance is often the best of all lessons.

Brain and Brawn

We believe reports about brain function benefits from physical activity.[5] Since Monty began a regular exercise program, his blood pressure and cardio fitness have improved. His energy, balance, and flexibility are all better. It seems in the first year of this latest fitness program that he fully recovered from heart surgery.

There is a caution, however. It is not easy to establish habits and follow them routinely. Because we are retired, we can devote more energy to this work. Keeping a digital diary makes a big difference because it is easy to use and keeps us focused on data and recordings.

We also credit our success to our daily thinking and modeling on how to live more fully. Keeping tightly to goals that can fluctuate daily requires never-ending consideration. It doesn't have to be much work, but consistency and daily consideration are essential.

Resolutions considered quarterly or annually are practically worthless. Active aging demands daily commitment. We know that thinking about specific goals often helps people to seek and accomplish improvements in performance. We can revise what we do when our weight stays stagnant, for instance, if we think about the day and plan how to make it all work, we will master the art of setting goals and sticking to them. Anything less, at least for us, is insufficient.

---

5   See: Amen, Daniel G. (1998). Change Your Brain Change Your Life.New York: Harmony Books, and Bredesen, Dale E. (2017). The End of Alzheimer's. New York:Penguin Random House Group.

Reflections on Physical Needs And Sleep

A good exercise regimen should lead to good sleep patterns. Both are important. If you have an active day filled with proper exercise, nutritious food, and a light supper, a good night's sleep usually follows. However, if you miss exercising, have several things go wrong, eat fast food or, perhaps, an overly spiced dinner and a few drinks late in the day and go to bed early or late, sleep—if it comes—is unlikely to be restful.

Getting a good night's sleep is essential. Insufficient sleep or poor-quality sleep can contribute to depression, attention and memory problems, excessive daytime sleepiness, and nighttime falls. Good sleep is vital to meet many of the brain's needs to integrate, consolidate, and ready itself for new rounds of daytime work, hunting, or whatever the modern person does.

We know that sleep is a vital part of our need for rest and recuperation.[6] Getting to bed after a long day, sleeping soundly, perhaps enjoying a few hours of dream time, is one of life's greatest pleasures. It is worthy of one's close attention to study Walker's book and do the many things which will aid in making sleep time into recovery and rejuvenation time.

We exercise early in the day to avoid interruption of sleep. Late afternoons can be the latest time to avoid sleep disruption. It is essential to find something you love to do and become even more passionate about doing it.

Keep Moving. Stay Active. Live Fully.

Sleep quality is also impacted by what we eat and when we eat it. Eat the best foods in moderate amounts at each meal. Keep track of your weight. Many check their weight daily to get an idea of what kinds

---

6   Walker, Matthew (2017). *Why We Sleep*. New York: Simon and Schuster.

of things push their weight up or down. Think of scenarios you want in your life, mentally model behavior that would lead to those scenarios, do the work, and reap the rewards. For example, we want to lose some weight, so we need to review what we eat and what we might change. When will we eat the new items? How will we obtain them? All of the what, who, when, how and where kinds of questions go into this process. Our toolkit chapter deals with these kinds of questions.

Meditate on your scenarios, do some visual imagery perhaps tasting the new food items. These types of mental exercise make change a part of yourself. So many things come to mind, including the real benefits to the brain, cognition, and memory, that it is difficult to summarize this chapter. However, a few things stand out. Do you sit a lot? Get up every hour and take a walk-around break; go outside, climb some stairs, or do some stretching or any movement. Keep moving.

Exercise is a significant driver in the quest for an active life filled with energy, fitness, joy and good sleep. It is essential for the individual to do the hard work, careful planning, and execution to age well. However, we also have to look out for each other. Couples know that if they don't care for themselves, the burden of their care will fall to their spouse, significant other, or companions and family. A duty we owe those people who may need our care is to be well enough, strong enough, and energetic enough to help when they require our care, attention, and love.

We all are in this together, and no one is sufficient by themselves for the task of growing old gracefully, with the vigor and excitement this golden age offers. Even with challenges aplenty, every day we see people going about their lives, making their days better as they work and play to connect more fully with life and its increasingly difficult-to-achieve pleasures.

Life's challenges continue even as the nature of life takes us through inevitable cycles. Those who are good stewards of their body, mind, and spirit are more likely to meet those challenges, giving it their best shot in tandem with friends and family. Did we do all of this correctly? No. However, we do better as we reflect on it while writing about it. We do better when we stay active, and active becomes more likely as we remind ourselves of the cost of inaction and the joy of feeling better and being more productive. How to live is a choice, and living actively is always better.

In this chapter, we explored physical fitness. There are other types of fitness coming up dealing with body, mind, and spirit. It is time to take a deep dive beyond movement and exercise into the subject of eating, nutrition, and the right fuels for our various needs.

CHAPTER TWO (Q&A)

1. **There are many recommendations for exercising. Is it really as simple as one approach fits everyone?**

Great question, and the answer is yes and no. Yes, the general message is that one should keep moving to stay fit and ward off diseases. The idea of eating a healthy amount of fresh fruits and vegetables and a moderate amount of proteins is general enough and will apply to everyone. Exercise like eating and taking medicines—they are all dose-dependent. Too much or too little may cause harm but not for everyone in precisely the same way. Moderation applies to all of these, and close monitoring of results is essential.

The problem is that we all start where we are now. Being obese and sedentary calls for strategies that will differ substantially from those needed by someone lean and fit. Also, a person recovering from a joint replacement will need specialized assistance to improve and move toward a more stable health status.

The warning to check with one's medical care team before beginning a new regimen of fitness and diet is good advice. We all must tailor what we do to any physical limitations at the outset of a new or renewed effort to optimize our health status. It is your health, and there is no escape from you playing a lead role in decision-making. However, there is much to read and learn in this area, and skilled professionals can be excellent guides. But YOUR intent to recover and reach new levels of fitness is the most critical; advice, counsel, and/or coaching from others are no replacement for YOUR dedication to YOUR health.

2. No doubt fitness is greatly prized over being unfit. How can I manage adding yet another chore into an already full day?

First, you must feel it's vital for you to tackle the motivation required to become fit, especially if you already feel overwhelmed. Being fit when older is critical, but age comes with years of living. Stay fit if you can, and if you're not healthy, get fit ASAP and stay that way. However, many of the diseases and infirmities of older persons begin very early. A few are genetic and begin at birth. Others are from sedentary habits formed over many years. [7]

If you want to start getting fit, the best time is NOW. Now you can take your first step. You might get up from reading and walk for five or ten minutes. Yes, just move. It is as simple as that. Begin that and make it a habit. Fitness opportunities come every hour of every day.

3. What else can I do?

Consider implementing a fitness agenda for ten minutes or so each morning. Ask what you can do TODAY to be more fit, eat better, or get more sleep. Do this EVERY DAY! Create plans to get fit to begin immediately; a resort vacation months away does very little good. You will be amazed at how easy it is to start the fitness journey if you do this every day. Ask yourself, *What am I going to eat today? Can I get in a visit with family or friends?* Perhaps you could have that late fish dinner but substitute the mashed potatoes and gravy with crispy Brussel sprouts. Maybe you could skip wine at a meal, eat a half hour earlier, and avoid stomach upset that often follows a sugary dessert. Ten minutes a day and a few things

---

7   See Li for in-depth coverage of many diseases and what can be done about them. Li, William W. (2019). *Eat to Beat Disease: The Body's Five Defense Systems and the Foods That Could Save Your Life.* New York: Grand Central Life and Style.

planned and done for TODAY! Hold that thought: do this daily, and you will succeed. It is as simple as it sounds.

You can also develop your own affirmative imagery or meditation for this time. We often repeat and reaffirm that TODAY is real. We can act on something today and today only on things that move our goals forward. Yesterday is gone, and time lost never returns. Tomorrow never really comes. Just the present is available to think, model, and act to make progress.

4. If I do planned workouts, what might work best?

Easy, work out five or six days a week. National recommendations run around thirty minutes a day. Our experts, readings, and experience consider that a good starting point but recommend going upwards to an hour a day.[8] But it isn't just the gym or workout time that you needed; continue the five to ten-minute brisk walking every hour or so. Movement is the key as well as getting the heart rate up a bit. Try to do this every day. Just moving hourly for five minutes or more seems a reasonable goal.

5. When and where is the best place to exercise?

Think first about what you can generally do in your home and workplace. Mimic your normal moves, and use them to strengthen yourself. Sitting down takes a lot of lower body strength. So, from time to time, rise slowly and sit slowly for five or ten times. Do you want to do some upper body work? Use your arms to lift your body from the chair. Without going anywhere, you get a workout. In the kitchen or bathroom, do some pushups using the counter. Taking stairs instead of using the elevator adds a good work out. Lifting

---

8   https://www.hhs.gov/fitness/be-active/physical-activity-guidelines-for.../index.html

hands and arms can also be done in ways that build capability or return to full functioning.

Retirement communities offer additional facilities for exercising. Community centers and fitness salons are widely available. If one wishes to improve their fitness, the issues of place, time, and equipment are not insurmountable barriers. In general, it is always a good idea to get a professional to assess one's movements; getting it right is a big part of improving one's performance. Right practice pays dividends; poor form can produce injuries.

6.   What are some of the main sources for good information on fitness and aging?

You can go to the Health and Human Services website for information on aging and on fitness. Physical activity is one of the essential things you can do for your health, it can help you to:

- Control weight
- Lower the risk of heart disease
- Lower the risk for type 2 diabetes and metabolic syndrome
- Lower the risk of some cancers
- Strengthen bones and muscles
- Improve mental health

Another general site for good information is: https://www.ncbi. nlm.nih.gov/. We also use other government web sites. No day goes by without one or more articles in our daily papers on wellness, fitness and diets. Many books appear in the book reviews as well. In the past couple of years articles on how to get more effective workouts by high intensity interval training. In our exercise classes we have been introduced into greater use of short intervals for keeping a muscle under tension. YouTube is a virtual university of videos on various techniques. We read, watch and try. Interval training has been adopted for aerobics as has time under tension for muscle exercise. Our search continues and we recommend that our readers do the same. Study and then trail and error, with a trainer where possible or gym assistant. Otherwise proceed with caution.

7. Many books provide footnotes to pin point the origin of ideas. Did you consider using footnotes for this purpose?

We did consider footnotes. In reality it is often difficult to pinpoint where one first encounters an idea. It can be equally difficult to pin down the original source of the idea. For example, our general knowledge of the reported fact that thousands of the baby boom generation is retiring weekly comes from many sources. Even the Social Security Administration quotes a research paper for their number even as they fail to note that the data comes from other sources. So we refer the reader to the best general source for that kind of information.

Another example of this difficulty is the question of the source for why beans are good sources of protein and ones recommended for replacing animal protein. Many of us born during the Great Depression were raised eating beans, not beef. The main use for cows was for milk. Moreover, most vegan and vegetarian writings recommend beans. Where did we first encounter that information? It really matter little for our purpose here and needs no citation.

8. Most of your active aging story begins in your late 40's. Were there other seminal books or events that propelled you in the direction of active aging?

We were both deeply impressed with the views of Abraham Maslow whose views helped shape our lives or was consistent with our earlier beliefs.[9] Whether his views shaped us or merely described us,

---

9   https://en.wikipedia.org/wiki/Maslow%27s_hierarchy_of_needs

go to his work for more insights on our drive to reach our highest potential, our belief in the human capacity for improvement and growth, and for our study of active aging instead of one or more of the afflictions impacting the lives of the elderly. Mihaly Csikszentmihalyi and Carl Rogers work has influenced our lives. Still there is another question, was it the work of these writers that accounts for our motivations or was it our motivations already extant that led us to those authors?

Where might we have begun noting authors and ideas. Monty went to Saturday morning movies where super heroes reigned. After he got his first paid part time job, he got the newest super hero comics from the drug store he passed on the way home from work. Later he read motivational books by Norman Vincent Peale and others which no doubt resonate still today. For Barbara, her role models were parents and teachers from her school.

Going deeper into sources of influence in our lives would require another book or two.

CHAPTER THREE

Nutrition: You Are What You Eat

Life is a one-person experiment
Study the science,
Experiment with the ideas
Pick ones that work for you

Early man's
Daily work was finding a meal
Food now is everywhere
Invitations to eat are endless
Choices matter
You choose, you decide

Our bounty is mountains of food always with us
Our curse is the abundance of food always with us
Our challenge, find the balance
Get a tad less than full

At each stage we live and learn
We produce, we consume
We work and play
Balance in all
We grow

What Is Nutrition?

Nutrition is that amount and quality of food essential to life. Our bodies take in food, which is then converted by complex processes into elements that are used to fuel cells. What we call our life is essentially a collection of cells doing the work of keeping us alive and doing what humans do.

Food for wild mammals—early humans included—was not always available 24/7, so the body functioned both in feast and in famine modes. Excess food converts into fat. Fat cells give up their fat when other needed nutrients are absent. Fat cells can burn as fuel. The biological mechanisms for these transformations are beyond this book, but it is a subject of much research and some controversy.

There is no one-size-fits-all strategy for sound nutrition. For some people, eating almost all vegetables, fruits, and nuts is essential. For others, a diet of mostly meat and potatoes is considered ideal. Still others think an intermediate course would be best. A single right approach for everyone may be unattainable because we likely are different in ways not yet fully understood. The human body can adapt to a variety of food sources.

The Standard American Diet (SAD) is three meals per day plus snacks, with foods high in sugar, fats, and salt. Since man's diet has been so much less predictable for eons that it is now, the amount of food needed per day is probably part myth and part cunning marketing plans to sell food. There is little doubt that this kind of assumption about the human need to eat so much eating contributes significantly to obesity in children and adults.

Most Americans rarely miss a meal and rarely go a day without food. For some, though, one meal a day is enough. After doing this research, we switched to often eating just two meals a day and no snacks. Before we retired, however, we fell squarely into the SAD diet that often consists of burgers, fries, and a shake often being one or more of an individual's daily meals (with sufficient calories in one meal to last a day). We probably did better because we knew more about what seemed to work personally for us and what did not. However, our work and habits did leave us vulnerable to a less-than-ideal diet, much as it does for most people.

When we lived in Tucson and were eating most of the time at home, our meals were similar, although Monty from time to time went on diets to lose weight. The diets varied, but the results were mostly the same: the diet would work, the weight would come off, and, after a while, the weight would come back. Barbara experienced less cycling, but her weight stayed on the higher side. Now in Kansas City, our meals are mostly ordered together but from a menu with many choices. So our diets have varied, and the results suggest two things. People who cook, eat, and live together will tend to have similar weight cycles, but when the diet can be tailored for each, the outcome for each can be different.

Nutrition is about nourishment for the body and how the body functions, survives, and thrives in our environment. It is a field of scientific study that connects the dots between food and what happens as it nourishes our bodies to make life possible. Government food policy is something of an unplanned experiment because national guidelines shift from time to time as new knowledge gains sway. For example, recommendations on fat consumption have gone from all to none to some and then to some kinds. Knowledge in many areas is evolving. Controversy continues over what is the best approach to nutrition. We guess that until we discover how to tailor our eating habits based on genetic predisposition, we will continue to find contradictions in our advice and predictions on what will work.

Nutritionists frequently recommend fresh vegetables, fruits, whole grains, legumes, nuts, meat, and fish. Humans can live off plants, nuts, and roots, or meat and fats; both show up in contemporary populations. While vegans do well enough without meat, the Inuit and other

Arctic tribes live primarily off blubber and meat from animals in the water and on land. Humans can go weeks or months without food but only days without water. We mainly are water creatures.

Humans today are not the hunter-gathers of our distant past. We buy in stores and cook at home or eat out. We eat on the run. Even at home, we eat more highly processed foods that use excess sugar and salt to improve the taste. The quest for ideal foods for the modern age runs along many tracks. The food industry seeks to enhance its products for public tastes. Nutritionists quest for the Holy Grail of a balanced diet that undergirds good health. Physicians and other scientists seek the underlying causes for all kinds of effects food has on chronic diseases. We study it to find out how to achieve high-level wellness, increase the likelihood of our health span equaling our life span, and on the excellent feeling of enjoying food and companionship that often accompanies eating.

Our Body Weight and Fitness Are Intertwined

Body weight is a vital aspect of being fit. One can be healthy and robust and still carry a lot of poundage and harmful excess fat. Alternately, one can be underweight and healthy or the opposite, underweight and in trouble. Nutrition is one of the critical ways of understanding how best to keep weight under control. Paying attention to eating is the key to body weight. For us, this is a constant challenge.

The good habits of paying attention to goals daily and acting in the present remain critical factors in getting one's eating patterns on a productive track. Only we can do it. The control of our body and our health is ours and ours alone. It doesn't rest with our parents or friends or our caregivers. It is squarely in our court. Regardless of how many times we fail, each of us alone has the power to take charge of what, when, and how we eat. For us, with choices at each meal, we each chose according to our individual taste and the dietary goals we have for the day. Each day's goals are predicated on each of our own sense of what we wish to achieve.

There is a significant caveat to this admonition. If one's partner lags or fails, it can harm the other. Fortunately, this works both ways. Doing the right things can have a positive impact on one's partner. In all things, balancing works best. However, in such places as our retirement eating programs, we can eat together but have special meals tailored to each person's diet plan and get more individual outcomes. This happens with us.

All too often, people go to one of two extremes when it comes to their health, and neither helps them achieve the objectives. Do you find yourself falling into one of these mindsets?

- I have complete control over my body, and staying healthy is merely a matter of mind over matter.
- No matter what I do, I will always be at the mercy of factors beyond my control, so why even try to regulate my eating?

We believe the properly framed question falls in middle ground: What can I do today to improve my health and perhaps contribute to better outcomes with the things that I have great difficulty controlling? At a recent lunch, for example, a desire for a burger was satisfied by leaving off the offered cheese and, instead of using the two slices of bread offered, tossing half the bun and eating the rest. It was a compromise. More than most days but less than it might have been and still very, very tasty!

Despite our cravings, nutrition is one area of our health over which most of us have substantial—if not complete—control. Let's look at how focusing on what we eat today can go a long way toward affecting how we live and feel tomorrow. What do we know?

Why Weight Control?

With few exceptions, obesity is a chronic condition for which we, as individuals, are the primary manager. Although others can help at times, our myriad of daily decisions are the primary help or hindrance in controlling this problem. By focusing on the individual's role in weight control, we are not sidestepping the issue of food being manufactured to appeal to taste sensations and marketing to promote excess consumption. This is a real issue. However, there remains an opportunity for control of some aspects of food consumption by individuals. We must each do what we can within the constraints of our environment.

Two in three Americans are overweight. If you don't think a little extra weight is a problem, try carrying around a couple of five-pound dumbbells the next time you are at the gym. Alternatively, put on a backpack with a comprehensive dictionary inside to get an idea of just what that weight does to your pace and posture.

Obesity is a significant issue, especially at advancing ages. Carrying extra weight probably was a major cause of stress fracture for Monty, and it can be a cause of discrimination in jobs. The US has laws which punish discrimination against people who employers do not think fit their ideal of employees. Obesity can be a burden on healthy bodily function. Chubbyness can wound an ego which absorbs the approbation from the general public and peers. In health care settings, workers with excessive weight can be viewed by patients as bad role models. Laws may protect employees but if obese health care staff are seen as a negative by patients, a medical practice can lose customers. It can be difficult to advise patients on dieting and exercise, for example, if the one advising seems to be living in contradiction of that advice.

We do not deny genetic influences nor are we dismissing the many food cues and sugar-laden temptations pushed by the food industry. We recognize the role of genetics in many aspects of biology and the workings of the endocrine system. We can take steps to control weight, but we have no control over the genes we inherit, although some of the things that cause the expression of the genes are controllable. In the future, we will know more about how to turn on and off many of the genes that might have contributed to Monty's stress fracture, but that is not possible now. We can act on weight, but working on gene expression is only now emerging with hints about ways to do this with lifestyle changes.

Our intent for weight control now is straightforward: much that is useful is within our control. We cannot deny that some of the outside forces contribute to our becoming addicted to sugar, alcohol, chocolate, and other things. However, at the base, the best way to stay on a correct course is by taking responsibility for our actions. Others cannot do this for us. Moreover, we should not dismiss the problem by blaming it on things outside our ability to control. Limit yourself to those things that you can command, monitor for new developments, and go on with life. Do today those things that you are best at doing.

Is calling for individual responsibility another way to blame the victim (ourselves in this instance)? Perhaps, but when there is uncertainty, we are all left with a decision—do something or nothing, and both are our decisions to make. We are building a more critical point here: whatever influences are most likely causing obesity, there are some that we can control. So we seek, and advise others to seek, control over what can be managed and go with that. Waiting for answers and solutions from others is a game we chose not to play.

We can all work with our natural endowments and use the best information available to manage our lives. As scientific knowledge advances, we hope to do a better job for ourselves in maintaining our health. Whatever else may cause a change in our health, ultimately we must deal with ourselves as we are, or, as a card player might say, we play the hand we have.

There are dozens of obvious reasons to keep weight under control. If you already have one or more chronic diseases, eating well and being physically active may help you better manage them. Some authorities argue that some chronic diseases can be reversed using dietary strategies.[10] We recommend studying these and considering them along with consultation with health care professionals. Good eating may also help you reduce high blood pressure, lower high cholesterol, and manage diabetes. How all of this works and how it might work for each individual is an unknown. Thus it becomes essential for each person to seek what seems best for themselves and to try it.

When making these decisions, even couples like us may lean in different directions. For Monty, some of the driving forces are based on family history. A brother of his died with Alzheimer's disease, a sister died of diabetes mellitus 2, and two other siblings died with hypertension and depression, which sometimes predicate Alzheimer's. So his search for clues, diet, and exercise regimens took on a more rigorous character. It has paid off. His weight the first year and a half dropped thirty-five pounds or so and has stayed lower for over a year. And his A1c, a diabetic marker, has fallen from pre-diabetic to normal in the 6.4 to 5.4 range. His mental state has gone from brain fog to good as ever, by his self-report.

Our biological control systems require a healthy balance of foods, without excess energy diverted to storing more fat than is typically required. What that balance needs to be is something that each of us must determine. Many competing theories about what works best make it even more critical for each of us to study our habits and try to find approaches that work for us.

---

10   Briley, Julie & Jackson, Courtney. (2016). *Food as Medicine Everyday: Reclaim Your Health With Whole Foods.* Ornish, Dean and Ornish, Anne. (2019). *UnDo It!: How Simple Lifestyle Changes Can Reverse Most Chronic Diseases.* New York: Penguin Random House Group. O'Keefe, James and O'Keefe, Joan. (2013). *Let Me Tell You a Story: Inspirational Stories for Health, Happiness and a Sexy Waist.* Kansas City: Andrews McMeel Publishing.

It is easy to agree with most recommendations for eating fresh food when available, consuming healthy portions, and not loading up on foods that seem to go straight to fat. Although the science behind all of this is never complete, we know enough to make a decision—reduce excess weight to a manageable level.

What Should We Eat?

The decision about what to eat depends on the interest of the recommending bodies; individuals have their favorites, and, like us, one must read, study, and actually try things that seem to fit to find the right balance. Governmental agencies that have studied these issues recommend a food regimen that stresses fruits, vegetables and nuts, eggs, lean meats, and fish. Over time as more research is done, the recommendations shift a bit. The many diet fads differ over time as well. We have tried many during these years of study and practice. Our finding is basically: all diets work and all diets fail. Even as this is written, new studies suggest variations on past themes and newer approaches based on one or another experts reading of the science and state of the art thinking. The debate about what is best, let alone ideal, continues. Our own choices vary from time to time.

Our personal approach today is more whole, plant-based foods, unprocessed organic, and locally grown when possible. In a retirement center, one can pick and choose among elements of meals on offer and find much of what one needs and desires. We have gravitated to less meat and dairy but not exclusively to a vegetarian diet but close.

In the early 1980s, we saw a push to reduce fat from our diets, because fat was considered a significant contributor to heart disease. Trans fats, which were created to add solidity to liquid fats and extend shelf life, got the worst ratings because they raised LDL cholesterol and lowered HDL, a double whammy. Trans fats lengthened the shelf life of food products and were a favored cooking oil for fast food, where they eventually were/are consumed along with the catfish and fries. The fats debates continue. Trans fats remain on the bad, bad lists.

Diets, Diets, Diets

We would enjoy writing about anything but dieting and extol the pleasures of eating a chocolate brownie with vanilla ice cream. However, here we are writing this book because excess weight and obesity are chronic problems that can be at least partially managed by the individual. And we are individuals who need to manage our weight. We are among the many people who try to seek the best balance in what we eat because, like fitness, obesity is a significant factor in almost every disease and cause of death studied.

Moreover, obesity management and an individual's success depend highly on the individual's efforts and tenacity. Study, intervention, and advice from others can help, but, ultimately, this is a chronic problem that must be self-managed. No doubt some of our issues are outside of our conscious control. No doubt the food industry makes it harder to sort things out. They can and do lead people astray with advertising. Still, we believe that the best approach is to enlist ourselves and other individuals in a quest to find the best balance for ourselves.

We can safely say that all diets succeed and all diets fail. We probably have tried them all, and, as many other people have experienced, the weight eventually makes its way back. There are many theories as to why we regain the weight, but, for us, the jury remains out. We read books and articles on the subject to help form our eating habits for living in a retirement community. We can have all our meals furnished, or we can prepare some at home. Most diet plans encourage preparing all meals at home, using precise measures, and calorically and content-specified ingredients. However, another strategy is needed when dining out.

From time to time, an article appears that compares and contrasts various approaches to dieting. The following list highlights much of what appears in the global media about nutrition:

- Some authors suggest the need to eat like our ancestors, who were hunters and gatherers that subsisted on animals and plants. Others go for the green colors of vegetables and the wonders of that carbohydrate bounty.

- More recently, we read about how our fat cells must be retrained to give up their bounty to produce molecules needed for energy production. Stop eating more carbo-hydrates, let the insulin from carbs become depleted, and fat metabolism will kick in and burn fat for energy,

- Fructose sugars are to be avoided, along with sugar sub-stitutes, which are notable hunger triggers.

- Sweets that come with their natural fibers are acceptable in moderation, in part because their textures cause the sugars to be released into the blood more slowly than refined sugars.

Bad Rap for Fats

Fats drew significant attention as the culprit in heart disease. For awhile, the consensus "settled" around fat as the primary cause of heart disease. Then came studies that seemed to show it was saturated fats; so no trans-fats were to be eaten, but other lesser, plant-based lipids were good. Sugar was also a contender for being a significant factor, but after the crowning of fat as the considerable risk, sugar receded. Science produces best theories and fits for the facts, but, as happens over time, others find aspects that don't fit the theories, and the search for the ulti-mate truth continues.

The debates about fat, sugars, and proteins need to consider fiber content. Generally, more is required. Fiber slows the impact of sugars in carbohydrates. Moreover, our digestive system and gut biome are both positively impacted by fibrous foods. Attention to diet needs to be more comprehensive than many popular diets suggest. There is growing evidence that our microbiome in the gut is a significant player in our weight cycles. Keep experimenting, and find what works for you. At this time, we offer no magic solutions.

So it is with dieting. Tomorrow is another day, and, hopefully, the approaches that you find to work for you will become ingrained habits. It seems there will always be surprises; the road is long and the setbacks many.

As with many other things in life, when one thing fails, plan another approach and begin again.

Sweet Temptations

Fructose derived from corn emerged as sugar of choice when fats were being shunned, late 1970,s early 1980,s. Just as fats in the diet were targeted as the major threats for heart disease. Inexpensive and abundant fructose from corn became a significant part of processed foods, which helped offset losses in taste when fat was removed. Thus, we entered a non-virtuous cycle of events. Carbohydrates with their higher sugar content substituted for fat became the norm, and weight went up instead of down, and then up, up, up.

Adding sugar to sodas no doubt has increased the calorie count of every drinker. Diet sodas have come under fire for cravings for sugar that might be stimulated by artificial sugars, as well as for the damage the chemicals in the soda might cause

Cutting out sugared drinks, reducing the use of most grain products, and getting higher quality protein, fats, and carbs from vegetables, berries, and nuts is the route we are taking. It seems to work. It also suits many of the general recommendations to eat fresh, whole foods and cut down on processed foods.

Fasting

An age-old habit of fasting for religious reasons shows that we can fast without harm, although consulting one's physician is always advisable.

The Mediterranean diet emerged in a region known for religious practices that often require fasting. We use fasting as a way to rebalance our input to keep the weight from bouncing back. Fasting that occasionally includes days with only two meals is becoming one of our ways to control weight. For us, fasting of some sort has become a regular feature of our lives. Several readers of drafts of this book have reported using fasting as part of their daily routines. It works.

Our diet now goes light on the use of sugar from carbohydrates. We continue to consume lots of vegetables for minerals and fiber as well as taste. Now the bread we eat is whole grain, nutty, and used sparingly, along with fibrous vegetables such as kale and carrots. Also, over time we are reducing the number of grain products, especially those that are heavily processed. Eating need not be unimaginative, but the temptation to leave the content to chance and food manufacturers is ill-advised. Confession: with chocolate cake, we sometimes add a scoop of vanilla ice cream. However, the next day, one meal of our two per day must be omitted. Don't neglect special events nor the makeup days later. Feast or famine is our balancing rule.

Salty Language

Salt often comes up as something to avoid in excess. We use it sparingly and rarely use it in restaurants or after cooking. We are aware that salt is an essential ingredient in mass-marketed, prepared foods. We also know that sugars from corn, which are cheap sugar, are added to mask extensive uses of salt. One of us, who is hypertensive, has long been leery of over-salting foods, so we shun manufactured foods most of the time.

Recommendations come and go and can nudge us in one direction or another. Each that seems appealing enough to consider should be carefully examined.

Dietary Recommendations

Which Recommendations Make Sense?

- Sort among the recommendations.
- Consult with professional advisors and friends, especially if what they are doing seems to keep them in good health.
- Finally, choose.
- The decision is always yours to make.

Putting It All Together

Now we will focus a bit more on what needs special attention in order for individuals to remain active as long as possible.

- Make a plan.
- Take action.
- Collect your data and assess to modify.
- Move ahead.

It is essential to first set specific goals for calories and types of foods needed to maintain the ideal body weight for ideal functioning. After that, one can craft a program to achieve those goals.

We caution you to remember that not all calories count the same. Some people assert that two quarts of ice cream have the same calories as a pint of beans and great servings of kale and nuts. There is a limited truth to that, but it is not true that mere calorie counts from such disparate foods best serve the body. Without fiber, the gut biome won't get fed, and a gut biome not fed from our food eats the gut; life has its imperatives. If you just feed your gut biome, say, sugar, your gut health can be a disaster. Eating whole foods with lots of fiber is essential, so merely counting calories is misleading at best and deceitful at worse. After years of experiencing diets where we lost a few pounds, but then it became difficult to lose more, we are leery of accepting the notion that just counting calories is meaningful. New Year's resolutions are the most problematic.

Many of our readings caution that the stabilizing mechanisms of the body will lower metabolism to keep energy use down and weight up. We carefully monitored calories and found that after a few weeks of some weight loss, we regain a pound or two. For example, Monty's weight went from 215 to 220 in a few days, so he began calorie restriction and partial fasting, eating within an 8 hour window. His weight went down after a week or so to 212 but within a few days of this it went back up to 215.

According to the calories-in, calories-out theory, weight should go down when fewer calories go in, but often it does not for days or weeks. The metabolism shifts instead so that it requires less food. Or the weight loss might be just a shift in water weight, which quickly goes up or down. Therefore, a 500-calorie per day deficit after a week becomes insufficient. Be patient, stay with the eating plan, and the weight will shift after a while. For Monty, if the wait seems too long, he moves to one big meal per day on alternate days for a week, and then his weight shifts downward. Calories in and calories out reigns as the best explanation, but it is a method that doesn't always work. No doubt some reasons it fails are related to the nutrients needed—a factor that is not taken into account by calorie counting.

For the Record

Valuable data is a significant asset in any qualified action plan. Keeping a record and going over it daily (perhaps more than once daily) is essential. It's great when weight goes according to plan. When it doesn't, the daily record may well help us understand what is happening. Several insights have occurred to us by consulting our food record:

- Did we add a new ingredient to the regular breakfast?
- Did these calories get moved from somewhere else?
- Did we inadvertently substitute something higher-calorie for a lower-calorie item?
- Did the body operate more efficiently?

Sometimes we don't know the answer to these questions, but the search proceeds, not for the specific answer but to discern any systemic failures that can be corrected. Good records, daily recording, daily reviews, and setting the regular schedule of things to eat and, when necessary, shifting around but keeping the overall goals steady is vital to success. For many, including us, weight management is as tough to deal with as any addiction, but unlike other addiction, you cannot abstain from eating forever and live. Weight must be monitored, managed, and controlled for life.

Where the Action Is

We have done several things to keep ourselves on track and to get back on track when our plans drift from the goals. The first important step is to pay attention each day and keep a record to review daily for opportunities to improve. With that, the following ideas come into play:

- Learn where you can cut a few calories.
- Consider eating whole wheat bread with whole grains added—or no bread at all.
- How about no desserts or just seasonal fresh fruits?
- Shaving serving sizes works for some.

Where we live, half orders or children's plates in restaurants cut calories without changing the balance of foods. One of our dieting approaches requires upping the fats consumed for a while and that, too, can be arranged. Life is about choice; choices we make daily. Drift is one of those choices.

The Natural Choice

- Eat the most natural foods you can. Green vegetables and fruit go to the head of our line.
- Tree nuts have the right vitamins and minerals, plus they are tasty and, for us, a daily treat. They are not calorie-free, however, so consume them prudently.
- Raw vegetables are better than frozen, frozen better than canned, and all of those are better than commercially prepared meals that are likely to be loaded with salt.

One significant advantage of natural foods is that fibers and trace nutrients are left intact with the food, not stripped out to meet the specifications manufacturers assume will please most customers.

Pause Before Seconds

Select a modest serving, don't go back for seconds, and decline to eat to satisfy others. A hormone in the lower intestine sends signals of satiation to the brain. It takes at least twenty minutes for consumed food to trigger those hormonal signals. So eat slowly and wait awhile before considering seconds. In our dining areas, not opting for dessert is the next hurdle.

Where Should You Start?

Pick the low-hanging fruit. Can you cut just one thing out of your regular diet? Perhaps dessert, which has lots of calories. Make deserts something very special, perhaps a once-a-week treat. Eat smaller portions.

One colleague would indulge in one spoon of ice cream, and only on rare occasions. Perhaps it should be bread or at least no white bread— just whole-grain if any, and then limit the amount. Stay with the process, whittling down as results come in, and persevere.

Monty began to eat berries for deserts, then for a special treat a small amount of nearly melted vanilla ice cream. All of these steps are required. Another natural choice it to ask for a half order of the meal to keep calories off the plate at the outset.

No Excuses

Avoid the easy way out that goes by the admonition of "if you go off a bit, just remember that it's only for one day and you can begin the next day again." That is true. However, if you use this excuse too often, results will flag and momentum lag. Miss a few good days and before you know it, you have stopped trying. This kind of failure can quickly occur when you don't take time to go over goals daily to get habits more ingrained so that they become automatic behavior. Automatic behaviors like always brushing teeth in the morning are superior to recent incantations of good intentions to change.

Today Is the Important Day

This process is an iterative process, day after day. It takes time and energy. It's simple but necessary. Habit formation is brainwork as well, so the process contributes to brain health. However, improvement requires more than mere repetition; it requires a continuing quest for growth. Development requires some ways to catch and correct the foods we consume. Data that you record and keep for yourself is one way to do that.

What we choose to eat, defines how our lives are lived out. We are what we eat or fail to eat, and what we eat can make life healthier. Our choices aren't everything, but they count, and they are uniquely ours to make.

CHAPTER THREE (Q&A)

1. **Are there things you learned during your study that were new to you?**

   In our early years together, we often ate out because our work schedules varied one from the other, and with both of us being full-time employees, eating out was our default option. Once we retired in Arizona, we ate at home most days and both enjoyed cooking. Our meals were things we generally agreed upon, although Monty dieted a lot and always seemed weight challenged. At home, we ate the same foods together and enjoyed similar cravings.

   Our move to a CCRC changed that dynamic. Now we eat most meals together, but we each order more according to our daily plans and individual taste. We can each follow eating habits different from the other. Also, it makes no difference in our relationship. When cooking for ourselves, this would not have been possible since we each share the entire meal.

2. **What are the significant challenges when eating plans diverge from each other?**

   That is much in the realm of eating that is challenging and required us to do a lot of study and experimentation. The current eating plan for Monty includes a longer-than-usual fast before the first meal—to noon or afterward after a 5 p.m. dinner. The calories count for his plan is much lower than expected, in part because with weight loss metabolism can drop, requiring fewer calories. Given such plans, we often eat mainly dinner on the same schedule. Many days we can also eat lunch together but with widely varying food choices.

Even as the foods we both prefer are whole-plant foods, our pattern of eating varies. Barbara eats a light breakfast and dinner and often skips lunch, while Monty skips breakfast and has a large salad for a late lunch and a lighter, earlier dinner.

3. How does exercise fit into your eating habits?

Weight control and exercise for fitness work together. The body needs to move for proper functioning. Excess weight adds unneeded burdens. Exercise alone, however, does not burn sufficient calories to lose much weight. But cut calories, especially the fats and sugars that add little nutritional value, and the weight will begin dropping. And fitness helps maintain weight control for dozens of reasons. Physical fitness is much easier for those who keep their weight under control.

4. Many find it hard to develop new habits, especially related to exercise and eating. How was it for you this time around?

The truth is that changing habits is difficult and takes far more time than any writer ever suggests. Still, it is essential. Frankly, developing new exercise habits has been easier than developing new eating habits. Also, with our meals being part of an institutional plan, it is much harder to pick among options and get the balance we want. So, frankly, the taste for sweets continues to cause both of problems. Sweets out of sight isn't wholly a banishment from the mind.

5. Since habits are hard to change, do you have any ideas to make the process work better?

Habits are difficult to change. But some practices become automatic behaviors that are done without using any particular prompts or willpower. These practices that can be moved from the conscious choice category to automatic are a big win. For instance, we worked on eating fewer flour products, bread mostly, first. It took a lot of willpower for many weeks, perhaps months, to get to the point where I just dismissed bread with little thought. Our willpower is now reserved for other things. We have also done much the same with sugar. We rarely have to think or mentally struggle to give up sweets. We use stevia when sweets still dominate some of our thinking.

Not having to struggle with such bread and sweets decisions reserves willpower for other hard and still-habituated choices we make daily.

6. Is there any one diet plan that you find most useful?

We use elements of many plans from time to time, depending on our daily goals. If the weight goes up a few pounds more than a four-pound range, we might adopt some fasting for a few weeks to get the weight back on the low side of the field. The thing we most fear is weight-creep, so daily monitoring guides our action when our weight slips.

At the time of this writing, we are zeroing in on a whole-food plant diet with little animal protein or dairy. Our journey is in progress.

7. When you say you do fasting, how does that work?

There are many ways to fast. There are solid reasons to do time-restricted eating. One such approach is to eat 500 calories per day for two days, with regular meals for the next five days. This is not strictly fasting, but it works to lose weight. Monty often skips one meal in the morning and has "breakfast" in the afternoon, thus fasting for sixteen to eighteen hours. Some fast for twenty-four to thirty hours between meals. We advise working with a medical professional for longer fasts than this. The fast helps to focus more on calories, and missing a meal for us means a 500-calorie or so restriction that day.[11]

8.   How about the use of carbohydrates, fats, and protein?

We use all three in rough proportions, but one-third each probably needs shifting to more fiber-rich carbohydrates and healthy plant-based fats. If we want fast weight loss, we might go high protein and fat for a week or two. But most days we eat all three—carbs, fats, and proteins—while paying close attention to getting more fiber. We also use probiotics and chia seeds and other fibrous items to keep our microbiome fed well.

The experts are out there with lots of reasons for many formulas. Study them, try them, think it through, and decide. We have no magic choice to offer. Experiment and pay attention to what is working for you. If anything comes through these pages, that is our message: study, research, and trust your own body to work for your best interest. Read the work of those doing population studies on nutrition and health. Also, consult your personal health professionals for their advice. Many are working for insights, and some are receiving them. However, what works for one of us may not for the other.

Doctors Weil, Ornish, Fung, Perlmutter, O'Keefe, Mercola, Lustig, Ludwig, Campbell, and many others have been read and re-read for ideas. The list could be longer but anyone reading these will have found each physician's touchstone knowledge and the research and reasoning for their recommendations.

---

11   Many of our readings are relevant to this general subject, some perhaps more than others. On Fasting see Fung's books including:Fung, Jason. (2016). *The Obesity Code: Unlocking the Secrets of Weight Loss.* Berkeley: Greystone Books.

9. Are there other questions lingering and being researched?

Many of the standards for nutrition are minimums set for the purpose of avoiding disease states. Optimal nutrition is rarely discussed and can be difficult for an individual to ascertain. Consider protein as an example. There are strong advocates for plant proteins being adequate, even superior to animal protein. Others insist that animal and fish proteins are superior, even essential, for optimal health. At our July 4th meal, we were served pork and chicken. We tried both of them for that occasion. And fresh Alaskan salmon is occasionally available at our retirement community, thus presenting an occasion for a deviation from more plant-based protein. There are no perfect approaches for all, and our knowledge is too skimpy for great certainty in this area.

Of the many subjects researched over the years, none has presented more challenges. It seems there is a perpetual debate over food. The science can be scarce. The National Institutes of Health budgets do not favor this line of inquiry to improve the health of the people. Food isn't patentable, thus it may not produce sufficient profit to justify private research funds and public funds tend to favor lines of research that can be commercialized later.

Our bets for the most likely area to lead to better health lies somewhere in the food and fitness areas, not in the finding of new elements that can be converted into medicines that are increasingly expensive. If we tried to list the authors whose writing on nutrition it would require re-listing the recommended reading list. More physician writers are mentioning food as medicine. We are inclined to agree with that direction, with one caveat: it should not require a professional degree to advise others on eating habits nor a physicians prescription for obtaining food.

CHAPTER FOUR

Intellectual Health: Use It or Lose It

You have useful skills, use them often
Want to try new things, do them
Get out, travel, keep moving
Like pets? get dogs, cats, birds, fish
Enjoy movement, dance, play
Have fun, laugh
Take a course, give
Listen to music, play an instrument
Cultivate an active mind

Live fully each day
When night comes, prepare to sleep
Sleep is rest time for body and mind
It is also dream time
Sleep brings new order,
creative connections,
more than we know

Stay fit, eat well, sooth your thoughts
After sleep begin your day refreshed
Awaken with insights into yesterday's puzzles

Cultivate your mental capacity

It's hard to turn on the television or surf the internet without seeing stories and advertising about maintaining physical and mental health during aging. Maintaining a well-functioning brain is critical to active aging.

Since we first retired in 1996, brain research has uncovered compelling evidence that the brain grows throughout the lifecycle, and it can adapt to changes in the body and mind by repurposing some of its circuits. Before those findings, we assumed that the brain was more fixed and unchanging. We thought it was only on a steady decline, with no hope of recovery and growth as one aged or lost some functions.

The brain consumes about 20 percent of our total daily calories, more than any other organ. As we age, the life, vibrancy, and functioning of this most vital organ looms large as both a great resource and, potentially, a great sorrow. Now knowing that the brain can grow and adapt to new uses, perhaps in ways yet undiscovered, makes it's fitness a condition worth careful consideration.

Here we focus on the brain, the organ in our heads that operates to receive sensations via other organs and then is able, via methods not well understood (especially by us), to use those inputs to create thoughts that we call "mind." Our brain is the site of our thoughts and our thinking, and it is the means by which we perceive the world around us. Recent research shows that our biome, the colonies of living cells inhabiting our gut, is in close contact with the brain and gets some of this credit as well. No doubt magnetic energies are impacting all of these systems as well; there are particles so small that they can travel through our bodies without touching, although their electrical impulses may well interact with those of the body, brain, and biome.

For the most part, however, all of these distinctions are outside the discussion in this chapter. We mention them here since in some circles such matters are central to understanding the role of humans in the universe. Here, we will stay with the issue more central to our thesis—active aging in a social context with our current state of knowledge.

One reason for calling this chapter "Intellectual Health" is to highlight the meaning that life has when we can think, communicate, create, and benefit from all body systems functioning effectively.

Much happens that is automatically controlled or influenced by the brain. Good cognition provides countless benefits. So explore, read, write, and create.

Many beliefs that years ago went unquestioned are now open to examination. Until the 1990's or so, it was believed that the brain could not grow new cells.[12] Now we know that the brain can grow new connections, it can self-repair, and it can repurpose when some parts fail. The mind can thrive when the body is kept fit with right foods that meet its needs. We do our fitness exercises to enhance overall health, brain health is at the top of our list of concerns.

There is a significant reason for wanting to keep the brain going. We need our mind working its wonders, providing us with endless opportunity to engage with life. In many ways, life is cognition and the mind is key to that vital function. Dementia is a significant health issue for the elderly. Lifespan after a diagnosis of Alzheimer's Disease ranges upwards of ten years. There are ways to cure some cases but not others. Some patients progress to a near total loss of function while others exhibit mild to moderate symptoms. Keeping active in body, mind, and

---

12   Most authors in the bibliography deal with this issues, some more than others. See especially: Mercola, Joseph. (2017). Fat for Fuel: A Revolutionary Diet to Combat Cancer, Boost Brain Power and Increase Your Energy - 2nd Edition. Enlightenment Now: The Case for Reason, Science, Humanism and Progress. Amen, Daniel G. (2015). Change Your Brain, Change Your Life: The Breakthrough Program for Conquering Anxiety, Depression, Obsessiveness, Lack of Focus, Anger, Memory Problems. New York: Harmony Books..

spirit are thought to ward off this form of decline or to at least mitigate such losses. The brain's capabilities are a gift, and its failure is a terrible thought to contemplate.

Sciences dealing with the brain are breaking new ground, gathering new insights almost daily. What we have gleaned for this book represents only our condensed knowledge about what we understand of the brain's functioning. No doubt additional insights will emerge that give new meaning or understanding to what we now know. Some insights will reverse old thinking, and others will reinforce why what we learned earlier is still the best insight. At this point, we believe that keeping the brain active is central to living an active life.

Physical Influences Mental

Physical activity stimulates the brain. As the working of the mind is improved, the quality of our lives is enhanced. Usually, cognitive activity is considered exercise for the brain. Our research suggests that physical activity also is highly essential for brain stimulation and growth. Body-mind connections are multiple, so here we will intertwine ideas about physical and cognitive activities that support brain health and functioning.

As we reviewed this area of knowledge, it quickly became obvious that research is expanding rapidly and that many myths about the brain are being challenged. It takes more than a few remarks to explore the many exciting findings and their implications for active aging.

The brain no longer is considered an organ that does not replace its cells with age.

As we shall see, the brain is a vital organ that is fully capable of growth and change throughout life.

Be Intellectually Active

How does the fact that the brain is a lifetime growth organ affect aging? We begin by examining the question of how the brain functions. What does it mean to be intellectually active? The most straightforward answer to this question is that the brain intends to think logically. It also performs other kinds of thinking—creative, procedural, humorous imaginings of the funniest things —to keep itself engaged. Learning new things often, challenging oneself to improve a skill, and more are about being intellectually active. It is important to test one's mind, sometimes pushing into areas of interest not fully explored, sometimes by taking up entirely new topics.

For Monty after retirement, his creative energies that had so long focused on management issues were deployed by observing nature and experimenting with various art forms. Barbara experimented with art and used her management skills to organize the neighborhood and build volunteer efforts. This book, a joint effort of ours, is also a brain challenge and fitness activity.

Watching TV might keep the brain going a bit, but it lacks the kind of challenge that working on improving our balance might have. However, this does not mean that TV is necessarily bad. It brings many good things, including the challenges to other forms of learning. After all, it can bring educational videos and lectures on subjects in which we need to improve our knowledge. The media that challenges us most seem the most logical ones to encourage brain growth. While we have had some wonderful travel experiences, documentaries and travel shows also greatly expand our knowledge of the world and the universe.

Keeping the mind in a growth mode seems the best approach to living well and staying mentally alert and engaged.

Emotions underlie much conscious thought. Feelings came long before earlier life forms combined to become human beings, as evolutionary theory teaches. Poets, writers, and other artists often speak of emotions in their gut, their heart, or in their bones as moving them to change expressions, make moves, find a different word or color. Our ability to see, touch, smell, and hear all inform our brain of the character of our environment.

Our gut introduces another long and varied surface for sampling and judging our most important exchanges with the outer world—our food, and its qualities. The gut has many connections to the brain; thus, it too is a vital aspect of our sensory armor and no doubt contributes significantly to the sensations that have their expression by and through the brain.

Our focus here is on the intellectual, or rational, aspects of our thinking. Chapters on social, psychological, and spiritual activity deal more with the emotional issue of thought and discourse, and aspects referred to as "speaking from the heart." It is convenient to separate these interrelated features, but by doing so, we do not intend to subscribe to any belief that considers that one is not influenced by the other. Also, there is emerging science that shows many influences of the gut biome on our brain, thinking, and emotions.

Purpose and Brain Function

We are thinking, rational, and emotional beings all at the same time. For instance, we believe that accomplishing most things often requires a purpose larger than mere self-satisfaction. Such a goal will be most meaningful if infused by a passion for making a difference through achieving it or contributing to such a cause. Some people exhibit a strong, early focus on their life purpose, while others may well discover their purpose as an evolution rather than a new revelation.

Purpose can be a powerful motivator. Having a life partner is one thing that can build a purpose in life. Each partner being present to aid the other is a significant contributor toward staying healthy. When Monty went through heart surgery, Barbara carried the load to support him and bear the primary responsibility for a substantial move to Kansas City. That experience and movement spurred our basic life design and rehabilitation efforts for us.

Purpose can help one harness the intellectual resources to get things done. Helping a child, a friend, or a cause can motivate us to pursue our personal goals a bit while putting energy into helping others. Our life purposes have shifted little between active working years and retirement: the health of people—that overarching goal for us and others—keeps us busy with many outlets. Barbara did some hospice work, organized neighbors for safety, and looked after many with illness or other problems. Monty taught a graduate course and help to organize a neighborhood association to deal with issues of land use and later standby emergency response capability via the development of a Community Emergency Response Team. Now that we are both in a CCRC, we engage in similar projects.

The purpose of caring for one another can be a powerful motivator for active aging. Maintaining brain health is straightforward when one knows that dementia or some other brain disease can arise at any time. We know that if we don't maintain our mental capabilities, it will not be possible to help loved ones. If either of us were to succumb to dementia, the other would be required to engage in many care projects. Thus, our life design project pays close attention to things that might delay or mitigate such a loss. Our life design book, *Active Aging*, is such a project.

We do not need to just read about mental loss; many at our age or younger are experiencing it where we live. Half of the US population over eighty-five are thought to have serious dementia issues. It happened to neighbors in Arizona and friends in Kansas City. It is a pandemic, not merely something someone gets. Our age cohort is at high risk. We are no exception. It is essential for us to take the steps we take to stay mentally active and fit.

Break the Age Stereotypes

There seems to be no age limit on growing intellectual skills and abilities, although the level of performance may slow. Doing things that challenge you to think is right for brain growth and maintenance of successful functioning. Like most physical activities, exercising your thinking capacity is presumed to be better than leaving your mind on idle or bouncing from one subject to another without any overarching goals or ambitions.

One of the stereotypes that needs to be put to rest forever is the one that says, "You can't teach an old dog new tricks." That is wrong. Learning may take more time, or it might be done more efficiently at other ages, but the brain of an older person may, in some ways, be able to learn new things. We are in the age category of Old Old at this point, but we still seek to grow and advance our knowledge in areas of interest. Admittedly, some things we are learning are things previously learned and forgotten. Of course, that happened when we were half our current age as well. We have a significant advantage now: we have learned many things over the years. Our memories remain active, so our reserves for tackling problems continue to be high.

One of the problems with age stereotypes is the fact that the stored memory and working knowledge for most of us are rarely used or sought by others. There are many reasons why this happens, but it means, in essence, that the world wastes a lot of talent, skills, and knowledge by encouraging early retirement and not finding ways to use more senior resources.

Don't Forget the Value of Sleep

Sleep plays many roles in our brain health. It's a time for rest from the distractions of current experiences that our active sensors are taking in. It seems that during sleep memories get sorted out, and questions that were raised during waking hours get more thorough vetting with answers sometimes available in dreams and at other times awakening us from sleep.

For years, Monty has found that "sleeping on a problem" and dreaming about it brings good, fit answers. Dreams can be states of thinking about which science so far has little to say. For us, especially Monty, the nightly deep sleeps and hours of dreaming are extremely productive with much too offer our daytime work and problem solving.

It seems likely that we can prime our brain to work on issues of importance. Athletes can prime themselves to imagine high levels of performance in their sport. Experiments have shown that imagery practiced while awake might help get bodily responses during surgery. Meditation and imagery exercises probably work on many things by implanting the memories in the brain.

Some thoughts just come from "out of the blue." Ever say or think "after sleeping on it" and follow with the idea that came long after the situation that had given rise to the question addressed? We often have such thoughts and know that it is our brain working to relate different memories and snippets of information that can be brought to bear on the question. Sometimes the thought will occur as if in a flash or seem to jump into conscious thought. That's what we often call our intuition. It comes without much conscious thinking about options.

On the other hand, there are ways to waste much mental energy. On the bottom tier, mindlessly watching sitcoms is a low-level activity. Writing letters or reading books is a step up, requiring some effort. And learning a new language presents a significant challenge. Taking up art in a serious way is also a significant stretch. Beginning a study of music, or at least learning a bit about the problems a violin player faces, for instance, illustrates what some do to achieve mastery in a subject or skill.

Use the mind productively while awake, and provide questions and desired states of being to aid the memory in finding ways forward to make one's life more productive, more comfortable, or just plain healthier! The mind is similar to many unexplored countries, waiting to be found and explored for good living. Ideas aplenty exist, but few of us get to explore most of them.

The bottom line: move out of your comfort zone and challenge yourself to gain an understanding of new things, knowledge, and skills.

Creative Thinking

Logic requires some structure and thinking that connects facts to conclusions. Our theory is that using the brain to read, write, sing, or dance will keep it growing connections. More and stronger relationships keep the mind working so it can do more things and more things well. Such a brain is essential to stave off the downward spiral associated with an aging body. Once the mind is challenged to do something, logical, analytical methods provide reliable guides to progress.

However, much of logic and logical processes seem to confine one to a universe of solutions that are relatively well known. There is another way to get answers—think out of the box, enter other cultures for novelty, and the like. In short, find a way to create new thinking.

Creative thinking challenges the brain to make new connections, or, as the *Star Trek* TV series said, go boldly where no man has gone before! The mind can be engaged in watching things without working to make connections logically. Creative thinking is natural when painting. Your mind can wander and let the colors and shapes light upon some thought that moves thinking along.

For us, moving from an apartment in Washington to a home adjacent to a national park wilderness area changed our entire visual field. Acres of desert plants, starry skies at night, and the howling barks of coyotes, cooing of doves, and buzz of insects excited every sense organ. Poetry chronicled the change and new hobbies and activities developed, including pottery, hiking, painting, and more. Putting ourselves in a new environment was an excellent stimulus for our creative endeavors. No doubt our brains were developing new connections, and the sensations reaching our brains were leading to new and innovative thoughts, emotions, and insight. We became more creative and in newly emerging fields of interest. At times, vivid dreams have a similar life-framing effect on our thinking and acting.

Creative thinking is intellectually stimulating, as is logical reasoning. Both are to be applauded in the challenge to remain active while aging. Many counselors recommend hobbies and volunteering to keep the mind busy. We did yoga, Tai Chi, spinning, and hiking along with pottery. There are no limits to what one might explore when it comes to making new connections, whether logically, intuitively, or by means yet to be discovered. The brain is a new frontier, with each intellect finding novelty in new directions for itself. Explorations of mental territory offer novel connections often leading to productive thoughts and new insights.

Our current creative thinking focus on this book. By researching and writing the book, is we are challenging ourselves to grow and exercise our brains. In this endeavor, we are expanding our knowledge by research and writing about our experiences. This writing is a continuation of our decades-long collaboration and exploration of how our life evolves. It also is a direct contributor to our own body and brain health.

CLARK

I'M FINISHED
WITH THE BOOK NOW!
I GUESS IT GOES
BACK TO MONEY
WHEN YOU FINISH
WITH IT.

ED

SHE WANTS TO READ IT
WHEN YOU FINISH IT.

Research and writing help clarify and expand our goals for exercise to mitigate the decline associated with age and to hedge against the systemic failures that lead to falls and broken bones.

Research greatly enhances and reinforces our vision of what fitness training can do for the brain and helps keep the body fit by staying active. These processes and projects feed on one another. The increase in mental functioning leads to more physical exercise, which, in turn, contributes to brain growth and improved psychological functioning.

Fueling the Brain

Research, writing, and dreaming keep the mind busy. These and more fuel imagination. These internal thoughts generated in the brain no doubt are food for the reasoning function. What we see, hear, and import from the external environment influences our thinking. We often are led in new and useful directions by creative thoughts and dreams. Ideas and uses of the mind come from a functioning brain.

The brain is fed sensations from both the outside and inside of the body. Our vision, hearing, and touch provide sensations that travel to the brain to create thoughts in our mind. Other feelings come from within the body, sent to the brain via the nervous system. This process also influences perception. We often think, "It was just a gut instinct," but then experienced no hesitation when it was acted upon. Brain and mind is often used as meaning the same thing. The mind results from the brains activity. Some thoughts and decisions are stimulus for other brain and body activity. One major name is given to such instinctual and seemingly impulse actions: consciousness.

Feeding the imagination makes logical reasoning far more meaningful. For example, when we watched a DVD about the art collections in the Louvre, Monty's painting gained exciting new directions. One particular video began with a discussion of Mona Lisa, a Da Vinci work considered by many to be his greatest masterpiece. In the foreground is the smooth, smiling face, while in the background lie the craggy mountains before which a large body of water dominates the surroundings.

This contrast was meaningful for Monty. Although his paintings of the night sky and wilderness experience—and now, city living—all yield similar results, the lines of human-made cities and the natural creation are opposites in tone and movement. In Da Vinci's *Mona Lisa*, that soft, enigmatic face contrasts sharply with the wilds of nature in the background. From this set of images, an important truth emerges: our external environment influences our inner landscape.

New research suggests that our mental imagery is mostly imagination, and only a small part results from outside input. Imagine that: we are dealing with mostly stored memory with only small amounts of real-time observation from the outside. The more we work on challenging our minds and exploring new learning opportunities, the higher our ability may become to have productive and meaningful thoughts. No doubt our many years spent studying many subjects in great depth stores our minds with ample perspectives to guide our thinking.

What should we do to keep our brains in good working order? Just thinking about how to age actively is a brain exercise. It is a way to grow even while aging. That growth will mitigate the forces of decline, making life more enjoyable. One of our preferred ways to learn about things is to visit cultures and systems different from our own. Early on, we took a course dealing with other health systems; traveled to Canada to see how their health system operates; and traveled to Britain, Sweden, Germany, and other places to help populate our brains with alternatives to our ways of doing things. Reading helps, and we often returned to educational programs to gain additional insights from alternative ways of thinking about things. By browsing, one can explore without physical travel—just mental travel and almost free of cost. Few days pass when we fail to find articles and books on subjects highlighted here. Today is no exception, as I bought another book highlighting food as the best medicine to aid the body in its effort to keep life going in the right direction.

Writing is one of our recommended brain exercises. It also addresses the larger question: Why be active? As will be seen in the chapters on spirituality and psychology, having a purpose in life pays dividends in doing things, in wanting to improve.

> **Motivation is the fuel for growth, which, in turn, is a boost to motivation to keep active. Working actively is itself part and parcel of a lifelong quest to grow and to serve.**

Mental efforts help the mind be agile, productive, and fully functioning as we age. Our leisure activities have an impact on the brain. Crossword puzzles and reading daily newspapers or professional journals and magazines, offer in-depth analysis of essential subjects challenging us to think about different aspects of events. For us, these things are natural and have been a part of our lives for a very long time. Not everyone's work and life experience included such reading. However, for everyone, retirement years are a great time to explore and dig into challenging reading for learning, growth, and great pleasure.

Resting the Brain

Meditation is, for many, a way to turn off or tune down the kind of restlessness that often characterizes the brain. Meditation states seem to slow the churn and allow the mind to register what comes while not engaging its content. We have practiced Tai Chi and yoga in the past for movement, and now we are beginning the Tai Chi practice again— this time for mindfulness and balance. All such methods have soothing mental and bodily strengthening elements.

To rest one needs to relive stress. To relieve stress, one simple breathing technique anyone can use is as follows: count to four as you breathe in; count to seven while holding the breath; and count to eight while exhaling. This works well for us. One of our fitness classes has adopted it as a closing exercise. When things get hectic, it often helps to do this about three times, slow things down, and then begin again.

Other techniques exist.[13] We seek comedy to relieve stress; or if in a meeting just tightening and releasing a muscle group helps. In conversations it is often enough just to show interest through facial expressions to relieve tensions. Find one or more, learn to use them, and take advantage of them to keep yourself on an even keel through rough times.

Never Too Late

The common objection "I am too old to start learning" is pure bunk. There is no magical age at which one is too old to learn. There might be a magical age for becoming a master violinist, but there isn't an age when one can't begin and make progress in exploring the world or the mind. For much of life and many fields of study and leisure, the doing of the activity is where the pleasure resides and where growth can occur. Reaching some arbitrary level of proficiency can be a goal but not a necessity for enjoying the journey and benefiting from it.

The theory is that an active mind will keep the brain mechanisms going. Science has found that the brain, like other parts of the body, can regenerate itself and grow. Not only does it regenerate itself, but it also can rearrange itself to take over functions lost through disease, disuse, or medical procedures. This ability to grow shows the elasticity of this vital organ. It also can expand in areas associated with some specialized

---

13   Kornfield, Jack. (2008). *Meditation for Beginners: Guided Meditation for Insight, Inner Clarity and Cultivating a Compassionate Heart.* Boulder: Sounds True.

knowledge as one increases skill and experience. We develop and adapt to our changing circumstances. No age limits on this seem to exist beyond the normal limits of lifespan, and that too depends in part on how we chose to conduct our lives.

Intellectual Pursuits Aid Active Aging

There are many reasons to consider active aging as a major life goal, one that drives long-term thinking and daily activities. Engaging in intellectual activities strengthens the mind, just as other exercises strengthen the brain and body. Therefore, reasoning about active aging is a journey and an intellectual exercise to stay mentally active and aware.

People who lead intellectually stimulating lives are more likely to be free of dementia. So keep moving and thinking!

Among the many joys of aging is the opportunity to explore things and places. Beginning a journey to keep the mind working and thinking in logical ways should be a lifelong pursuit. It is for us. As we read, the world becomes an open book. With books available in digital form, a whim can become a reality in the few minutes it takes to order and receive delivery of a book. Such easy access can be hard on the budget, but it makes research and reading easy. In minutes, one has access to the world's knowledge. For someone with a more limited budget, the public library can offer many of the same benefits.

Whatever might lead to becoming more active seems likely to be a benefit. For the painter, a visit to an artist's studio or art exhibit can provide great pleasure and offers insights for one's creative endeavors. For a dedicated golfer, a book on exercise written by a golf professional will be superior to one done by a pianist.

Some societal advances are equal-opportunity resources. Computers have revolutionized learning opportunities. We now have almost all of the world's libraries at our fingertips. Access is becoming faster every day. These machines have opened every library in the world to exploration. If you don't have a computer, use one at the local library. Knowledge at your fingertips grows evermore present. Opportunities to explore are boundless.

It is pleasant to exchange ideas, and social interaction has its benefits for the brain, mind, and spiritual development. For some, writing is another great gift to one's knowledge. As writers ourselves, we're not surprised to hear other writers say, "I don't know what I think until I write it." This is another example of how expressing oneself in an external format aids learning, thinking, and growing. Mental modeling works, but getting things into writing works better.

Why, one might ask, would the explication of an idea in writing aid in the perfection of the concept? Perhaps the idea, once thought of, is amorphous, less than complete, and subject to shifting as one mulls its meaning. To write the idea, the brain mechanisms communicate with the fingers on the computer keyboard. Doing this engages feedback loops and no doubt other aspects of the brain that are needed to do the work, such as stored memories that tell us how to punctuate the things written. In short, many aspects of the brain engage in the process, so the mental imagery of the idea or model takes on stronger connections.

As one ruminates about ideas, complex interactions among regions of the brains occur; and through these exchanges the idea gains greater detail and nuance. Writing forces the development of ideas into more elaborate structures. Ruminating over an idea seems puny when thinking of the complexity of the brain and the concept of the mind, its operation, and change. But why not at times slow one's reading and linger over a word or phrase? Prose can easily become as potent as poetry if read with intent and curiosity.

Writing with computers can be fascinating. Words, phrases, and sentences appear, and the mind can usually instantly recognize whether they make sense or not. It's like having a mirror to the mind right there, checking each idea or thought. Reading one's writing aloud brings another great sensing tool into play and will ferret out nuances that the writer might want to include and help recognize things that will not work when communicating with others.

Of course, there are downsides to writing with computers. Sometimes the computer will substitute the wrong word, using a word that's correct structurally and grammatically for the sentence but wrong for the meaning. Nothing is without some challenge.

Mental Challenges Exist at Every Stage of Aging

The first big step in thinking through the issues of active aging is to focus on just what it means to you to age actively. For someone at twenty, such a question likely would be dismissed. It just isn't the essential thing to think about at that age. However, many things one needs to consider for active aging are, in fact, things that, if begun as a child, would be the most effective, such as eating fresh whole foods, getting exercise, and developing the habits that keep one fit and healthy. Ideally, one might develop a life plan at a young age that including active aging.

We both began work and study habits early but not fitness activities. Study and work is the pattern for our lives, with little thought of sports. In college, Monty worked to pay his way and support a growing family, and Barbara worked nights as a nurse while earning an undergraduate degree to support her work. Work for both of us required lots of moving around, so that was it—no sports for recreation.

What one didn't do in the past is relevant only in helping determine where to start today, in the present, on any path one chooses to take. The fact that we had no sporting experience leaves us with the need to develop a new level of fitness and then to find a sport that makes growth and improvement more likely. For us, walking seems the most obvious choice. Speed walking might be a second step. In our balance classes, meant more to avoid falls, we occasionally pass a basketball back and forth. Volleyball is another sport that might move us along the fitness trail and keep the mind more attuned and prepared for sudden movements—a crucial ability for staying upright.

Someone in their forties, when childbearing becomes less likely, might be a bit more likely to concern themselves with active aging. Because the half-century of life looms just ten years ahead, questions of how long to work, how to ensure that savings will be sufficient, and how to live after their working years will either creep into consciousness or financial planners will ask about plans and expectations.

Financing the Dream

Our financial planning for the future began in our late-forties. At that point, it was simple: enroll in all pension plans available, learn to live on less than we earned, and pay down our debt. As academics on contract for nine months, we could gain an additional few months of paid work to supplement modest salaries by finding grants or research support. We had seventeen years to secure a retirement future with anything more than social security. With no savings and college cost for children looming, the subject was a serious concern. Our attitude toward consumption was to live below the level of our earning and to allocate some to saving for emergencies and retirement. We coupled modest living and saving with our deeply engrained habits of education and work to provide resources for our long-term needs. While our challenge was not unusual, it was never easy. However, when possible, an earlier start on saving and investing is highly recommended.

Financial planning came up again as we reached our mid-fifties and retirement years were not far out. We had both saved via our educational pensions systems, which vested from day one. Our careers, while going well, had horizons beyond which we would need to refresh our knowledge and skill base again or move into jobs that did not require cutting-edge abilities as our work did at the time. So we turned to pension experts for working models. Judging from the retirement planning models, five or six years of maximizing our savings would provide for a timeline of retiring in our early sixties. Our thoughts were not to quit work entirely but to transition to jobs that did not require extensive travel and left more time for leisure and becoming settled in one community. A sometimes-fickle job market for seniors is a dicey thing upon which to depend, so we doubled down on work.

However, as we aged so did the client base we had cultivated. In order to keep up, we needed to expand our base, and that meant greater effort to build some new services to offer or find a new cohort of client possibilities. We chose to renew our policy credentials by moving to Washington, DC, to participate in more national meetings where we also could contact more potential clients.

While good savings and well-paying jobs count for a lot in terms of options for living, it is important to remember that an active aging lifestyle can be done on a wide variety of budgets. Friendships can be cultivated at any age or income; libraries can supply any book one might want to read; and walking outdoors or in malls is open to one and all. But to have the widest range of choices, you should get a good education, invest in your own capabilities, save all along the way, and keep working as long as possible. Here's the most important truth:

Hard work and long years of challenge provide great benefits to good health and long life.

Staying active is most likely to lead to a healthy life. This book is a product of professional work done during the ages of eighty-three to eighty-six, and eighty-five to eighty-eight respectively, with plans for more work following this activity.

Writing about thinking reminds us of the questions that accompany most quests for knowledge and insight.

- Is it something important to me?
- In short, does this matter, and is it worth pursuing?
- Is it my highest priority now?

The character James Donavan in the movie *Bridge of Spies* often said to Rudolph Able, the Russian spy, "Aren't you worried?" Able always replied, "Would it make any difference if I were?" Would it make a difference in your life if you gave the issue of active aging much thought? Unlike the answer Able gave, the answer is a resounding, "Yes, it would matter." You will have a fuller life. Your health likely will be better, the years you have will see less pain, and you will have more years of life as well. We still reap new benefits from this thinking. Even as this book is almost finished, there is a new one coming into view on creations and the use of poetry and painting. Active minds are creative minds. Stoke your creative thinking, doing so will help to light the way to greater opportunity. One might reasonably ask, "don't you take time out just for fun?" We do but still we too ask that question from time to time. For example, we noticed an article in today's online newspaper about the top 50 tv series. Thinking of this question of fun, we read the article and found none to our liking. So life goes, our reading and watching runs more to documentaries, novels and issues of health, fitness and life purpose.

In our daily lives, the following questions can be our best ones to ask: What is important? Does it matter? Is it worth pursuing? Such issues are important to ask and for that reason alone were featured in the *Bridge of Spies*. For our purposes, health problems often are of paramount importance and take precedence.

We value questions that invite us to use our minds to imagine alternative ways of seeing things, doing things, learning, and the like. This keeps our minds challenged to reformulate questions and possible answers that will be more amenable to action, change, and growth. Science often gives us answers that lead to new questions and changes in how we view the world. Mental challenges lead to exploration, and exploration leads to growth of mental capacity.

Good thinking, like science, is more a journey than a destination.

Things generally seem settled in life until more insight or a new paradigm comes along. The mind is humanity's tool to understanding, to building, growing, and no less so to finding the best ways to remain active intellectually as we age.

Many things go into determining what happens in our lives. We are forever challenged to come up with logical ways to proceed, and we do. When we make mistakes, we figure out why and try again, often in different ways until something moves us along. In short, keeping the brain healthy and mind going is a process. There is no fixed and eternal answer but rather a process of unveiling and change. One makes judgments and moves along. If we retain our curiosity and a tendency to seek actionable solutions, we can be a good learner and active.

A Focus on Purpose Aids Navigation on Winding Roads

Our thinking about how to age actively took twists and turns. Thinking about the mental aspects of active aging can help, but it also is a personal quest that goes beyond the challenges faced by merely aging more productively. It is essential to engage your sense of self, your feeling self, or, as some say, to lead with your heart. It is difficult to embark on thinking about behavioral changes without a feeling that difference can help, that change is possible, and that change can happen with persistence and hard work.

By focusing on the rational side of intellectual pursuits, we are almost by definition not exploring another, perhaps more important, aspect—feelings and intuitive senses that often guide our actions. Frankly, we know little about how intuition works. We are believers that it exists and is important but have no idea of just how to improve it. Listen to your heart! What does your gut tell you? What is it that moves you to quick action before knowing in a conscious sense just why you are doing something? This element of our body-mind-spirit simply is, and one needs to acknowledge that and use it.

Monty has long recognized that he can often come up with better insights after a night of sleep. He also knows that sometimes he can't explain at the time just what moved him to act, but knows that he does follow senses that are not at all available by his more rational processes. We all have these senses. We don't cover this idea in detail, but listen to your heart, your gut, and those insights that come after or during meditation or sleep. Learn to trust yourself.

How often do we say, "my gut reaction" got my attention and directed my response? Or, "It was just a gut reaction!" Billions of microbes inhabit our bodies, and our gut connects to the brain. Maybe those "heartfelt" things are also gut-felt and gut-acted -upon feelings. The gut biome performs so many vital functions that it is entirely logical for signaling to occur between the mind and gut centers, thus creating something of a co-cognition person. We have evolved along with these life companions. It is our shared destiny that is at stake, so do not ignore this emerging area of scientific concern and attention.

The brain can grow and change. Stumbles are first learning opportunities. Believe this and grow; if you don't believe it, fake it until you do understand! It works.

A personal quest for excellence in any life pursuit, a passion for a cause that drives us, helps immensely. For us, it is now, in part, to be able to care for each other in tough times and the unknowns of our now not-so-distant future. We have a book to write, paintings to paint, projects to finish, other challenges yet to be found. For others, it is sufficient to be able to walk the halls to dinner or to walk or climb stairs for a seat at a symphony. It helps to have a stronger purpose in life to sufficiently motivate yourself to do the hard work of maintaining fitness. Many young people are urged to find a purpose and pursue it for life. That works for some, but for others, it means leading a life of search, exploration, and, over time, finding underlying themes to their lives that reveal purpose.

What if you don't have a definite purpose in life? Think deeply about what is important to you now and how you might enhance your ability to deal with it. Then get better at doing what matters to you. Life is a lot like a fast-flowing stream. Consider how well a boat does in such a creek without a rudder. It drifts and often runs aground or capsizes when it hits a rock, tree, or a turning point. Find a purpose and guide your life through the stream of consciousness.

"Seek, and you shall find" is a substantial universal truth. When progress is glacially slow, some people persevere in efforts to mitigate decline to maintain their independence in life. Some are always on the move. Just yesterday we dined with a person who works out a lot. Before most of us finished the meal, he went off to do some stair climbing. Some have a built-in activity generator that needs no priming. For others, sitting longer, having dessert, and then taking elevators is more the norm. For those who require a more thoughtful and planned approach, this book may help. For those who are self starters, it will provide ideas to explore. Most of us have people in our lives who need help being active, so share it with them.

Keep moving. Make every day an opportunity to succeed. Moving on goals every day applies equally to other aspects of life, including eating well, keeping your social and professional networks fresh and up to date, maintaining strong family ties, and saving for that inevitable rainy day. If it doesn't happen naturally, work on habits to make it so.

Improvement (and Myths to Avoid)

We have long subscribed to the idea that engagement in learning throughout life is essential. It is also important to continually seek to improve the things one routinely does. Those who are best at something always seem to get better over time.

Improvement requires a commitment to use our energy and talents to become better at whatever we do. Improving the performance of our bodies and brains should be among our highest goals in life. Without high-performing body and mind, all other goals become more difficult to achieve. Whatever our commitment to other things, our performance will depend on how well we prepare physically and mentally for work or play. Among those things we need to learn more about is nutrition—what keeps us well and our cells functioning correctly and providing us with the positive energy required for a full and healthy life.

Two of the most potent untruths and too easy excuses are "I can't" and "I'm not good at it." When you say these things to yourself, know that it is simply not true, and while they are potent falsehoods, they never were real. Does that mean that everyone can do everything? No, but it means that if you work daily toward a change goal, given where you are at present, you can improve.

If you want to grow in your skills and abilities beyond that which you can get just by reading, imagination, and practice, set goals for improvement, find good ideas, keep track of what you are doing, and use data to improve. From time to time—or for some, all the time—use an expert trainer to guide, monitor, and help set improvement goals.

An expert is just someone who knows a lot more than you do about the subject and can guide you in improving your skills and knowledge.

If you are not a reader, ask a friend about their favorite book and read that. Discuss the book with a friend. Learn more of what they might have learned or like about the book and why. Do this, and you are on your way to becoming a good reader. If you are not satisfied with the first book, seek guidance or discuss your interest with a librarian. It is incredible how much help is out there for someone who wants to use reading as a cognitive exercise. However, reading books is so much more than training; it is an opportunity to journey into other worlds, savor strange and exotic foods, or smell the air of the open sea.

Just Imagine

One can stimulate the imagination in so many ways. The ability of the mind to IMAGINE things is an unusual gift, a treasure, our most valuable possession. It can fuel our inner world in so many ways. Please do everything you can to enhance this mental ability: use it daily, feed it ideas, and keep the biological brain on an even keel with exercise and proper nutrition.

Keep the brain at peak performance and the mind ready for adventure. Then be prepared—you may begin to get the itch to travel, take up a hobby, or get to know a new language. Learning new things can become a pleasant and useful addition to life. Substantial improvement can be gained just by walking more. Getting better may take coaching, research, reading, looking, listening, and lots of practice. So it is with cognitive activities. Moreover, becoming an expert means getting feedback on how you are doing something in order to learn the most efficient approach and practice it. Then it means finding the next improvement you can make. Your goals should guide how far you want to go. Nature may well set some limits, but rarely does it inhibit people from getting better at their work, sports, and hobbies. The theory that it takes ten thousand hours to become an expert is probably true for some specific set of skills under certain circumstances, but it isn't a universal rule.

The same reasoning we use for sports applies to mental efforts. Want to become a more-serious reader? Go to a few lectures by authors. Read their books beforehand and then ask them about aspects of it you find interesting or puzzling. If that doesn't work, try C-SPAN on cable networks. It's a free channel and has weekends devoted to authors and books. An entire world of information awaits to help anyone develop and become a more discerning and capable reader. Along the way, you also can work on your writing. Learning is an excellent way to expand your interests in life and to encounter enjoyment beyond words.

Perfect Practice Makes Perfect

Doing things in the best way and practicing that method will lead to progress and improvement. The quest for finding the best way to do something is the key to overcoming another myth: practice makes perfect. In reality, practicing in better ways and continuing to improve is what makes for perfection.

In any given sport or profession, there will always be opportunities for creating new methods and making breakthroughs. Rising to higher levels of skill means doing deliberate practice and then getting good coaching and feedback on performance. Keep challenging yourself to do things even better.

Consider music. If you want to learn to play an instrument, it would help if you began with a teacher, a coach who gets you started to master the basics. Get better at it, and it will eventually be essential for you to get a new trainer whose skills can move you to a higher level. Each coach can handle one or two degrees of ability. Beyond that means shifting gears and moving to the next challenge.

This advice applies to more than physical fitness, reading, or piano playing. Carpenters, plumbers and electricians have technical schools and apprenticeships to do much the same. Although some things require standards and the ability to do what the masters do, many physical and mental activities can be made more accessible from the ideas and methods gleaned from studying experts in their field. As you study such purposes, you will strengthen your mind and in the process learn more about how to make other aspects of life more meaningful and useful. Many people who have achieved significant things in their fields of interest share their insights through books. Find those books, read them, and gain insights from others who have traveled the path you seek to take—learning comes from those who share their stories.

Some Olympic athletes have experienced injuries that interfered with their practice. By mentally modeling and thus imagining performing the movements required for their sport, they were able to enter the competition and perform well even without the usual physical training. The mind interacts with the body and the body with the mental enactment of their sport. Although what, exactly, is happening may not be known in a strictly scientific manner, the techniques used are often known. Our growing knowledge of advances in science spurred our interest in making the connection between the physical movements of the body and their impact on the mind.

Diverse Stimulation

It's always fascinating to watch people in other disciplines and occupations go about their work. Many role models are available in each of our lives if we take the time to learn about their journeys. Sometimes it's a teacher or co-worker. Or someone you wouldn't expect to learn from. Monty learned a lot about panhandling when approached by a man seeking money for breakfast. Instead of giving him money, they had breakfast together as this man shared his techniques for living by begging. Most days still offer opportunities to learn. In our retirement living, neighbors share their stories daily.

Work life and cognitive development go hand in hand. Learning is a big part of work if you want to master an art or craft.

If you learn how to learn, then growth is more likely.

Learning to learn means being systematic about your search for meaning. Going deeper and broader in your area of expertise helps. For us, as academics and later as consultants, that meant studying health-care systems other than our own. Some we read about. Occasionally, we traveled to other countries for study and field trips. One can learn much from learning about how different cultures do things. We learned much from our visits to Mexico, Denmark, Italy, Canada, Ireland, Great Britain, Belgium, Sweden, Germany, Israel, and China. Even now we have a bucket list for other places we would like to visit.

Broaden Your Horizons

You can learn a lot by getting outside of your backyard and visiting other cultures for ideas and personal growth. After one of these visits, it became clear to us that tackling the problems of cost, efficiency, and quality of health service was putting the problem backward. It was more likely that much of what was needed was in the control of the individual, and it is there that the significant interventions were required.

What does having the individual involved mean? Much of what makes for good health is in the hands of the individual—the mom, the dad, the school administrator, the officials who lay down rules and decide what works best. One story we heard was that of a coach who decided that just being on a sports team standing inactive on the side-lines was a waste of time. He nudged his school to require fitness time daily for everyone, with sports an additional option. Once the program was initiated, classroom performance and test scores also improved! So physical activity that challenges human performance can improve cognitive performance. This is an excellent example of mind and body connectedness. Keep moving, work out, push the cardio system on a routine basis, and body and mind performance will improve.

Actually, every day that one doesn't do the things that would promote fitness and well-being is a missed opportunity. But like the sports not started, they simply are not relevant or worth time regretting.

Today, opportunity exists to begin again. Take it!

You can access a great deal of cognitive challenge not just by reading and going to school but also by finding ways to apply learning to daily life. This book is an example. To write it, we needed to do research to find out what was evolving in the quest for knowledge in the areas we thought were important for active aging. This required researching, reading, absorbing and analyzing how the things being discovered affected our lives, and then finding a way to incorporate the new learning into our daily routines. And, further, it involved determining how to communicate it to others. More importantly, we tried the various ideas to see how they worked for us.

Writing this book is a cognitive challenge, a case study in active aging. This long-held quest for how-to's and whys of active aging is now itself a prime example of active aging. Many people have stories, and in the telling of those stories and teasing out the life lessons, they will be contributing to their own ability to successfully navigate the challenges of aging healthily. Reading about and listening to the stories of others enhances our lives.

Now living in a retirement community, we continue our work of observing and thinking about how to improve the delivery of health services to benefit people in their communities. In particular, we are deeply involved in thinking about how to optimize our own lives in the city at an advanced age.

For example, before arriving at our current home, it seemed that to move into such a community would be like going to a nursing home. However, we now know older people here who have varying degrees of disability and are actively engaged in doing powerful things. We encounter many who remain active—a few at paid jobs, some serving as longtime volunteers, a few into active sports, and many dedicated bridge players. How people age varies widely, but the most active are the ones most likely to have the most physically demanding activities in their life. However, there is an equally good example of those whose most potent moments are at the bridge tables. Our goal is to find ways to optimize our opportunities to stay active.

Things to Remember

The literature on aging is replete with suggestions for being active and maintaining health with proper physical, mental, psychological, and social functioning while growing older. Population trends indicate that lifespans are getting longer, which puts more people at risk of a rocky decline in their last years. We need general strength training and practice using specific muscles and reflexes to injuries. Why? Strengthening the essential muscles and related tissues is important. In addition doing the movements refreshes the brain's memory of them, making it less likely to fail to move quickly enough to right oneself from an awkward turn. Each of the many moves made daily can be the object of training to lessen the likelihood of injury and successfully navigating our daily lives.

A few tips seem to be in order:

- Lightweight lifting and balance classes help us retain muscle memory required for awkward moments, such as the sudden movement or the twist we might take to avoid colliding with someone else. Flexibility and balance are critical at such times. Those who fail to maintain such muscle memories end up with broken hips or worse outcomes.
- The brain needs frequent reminders of essential muscles and how they must be coordinated to function effectively. Falls are constant threats to older persons, and the best way to avoid them is to exercise the muscle groups that, when weak, can fail to function effectively when some adverse event occurs.
- Are you not lifting your foot high enough? Didn't see that change of elevation? The brain has lost its sharp edge for the quick response needed. The brain needs refreshing, just like the muscle groups that do the work.

Hard evidence is accumulating that brain exercises such as reading and challenging your brain's abilities can help prevent or slow dementia of various kinds.[14] The evidence is sufficient to recommend doing exercises routinely for life, because as yet no studies show it doesn't help, nor does it harm the brain. Learning new things presents the kinds of challenges the brain needs for exercise. Chess, bridge, and other games are useful. Running, jogging, and other fitness exercises also help. [15]seem to be less susceptible to mental decline.

Inner Motivation

Dedication to improved performance is associated with self-directed learners. These are the people who seek advice. They read widely and

---

14   Bredesen, Dale E. (2017). *The End of Alzheimer's: The First Program to Prevent and Reverse Cognitive Decline.* New York: Penguin Random House Group.
15   See this article and others on government web sites:https://www.ncbi.nlm.nih.gov/pmc/articles/PMC4435622/

find ways to train themselves to perform at a higher level. They can handle more difficult challenges. They can conquer a fear of heights, lose the weight to help keep blood pressure lower, and do the harder things to remain healthy or regain health after accidents and medical procedures. Practice helps, but without finding ways to improve execution or push to higher levels, one doesn't get better at things and even may get worse.

Seek to improve your performance. It is in the quest to do better that we grow.

In our opinion retirement ages will increase for two big reasons: (1) individual health will be better because continuing active lives improves health, and (2) it takes far more societal resources to support people who don't work and contribute to their cost of living. Either way, it is essential to lay the base of fitness and activity to sustain a healthy life.

Development of a passion for one or more sports (playing them, not just watching) helps to stimulate the mind and motivate one to stay engaged with an active lifestyle. Excelling at any physical (or mental) activity requires a foundation of overall fitness. Being a great player in any sport now means regularly working out the entire body. Each mental activity requires special and general preparation and functioning. Excelling at the piano, for example, is different from playing chess. Exploring ancient texts requires language studies and immersion in cultures where the ancient language is dominant. Physically fit scholars have a better shot at excelling at the full range of activities than those who are unfit. On the flip side, someone can be highly fit physically but not do well in a scholarly discipline if that work has not also been the subject of more intense study and improvement.

The good life requires not only balance but also growth and excellence in more than just the physical or cognitive spheres. Are there exceptions to this rule? Yes, in many fields, people with significant handicaps and setbacks in their lives have attained great achievements. Also there are those who are models of physical fitness who have not improved their use of their mental abilities.

The brain can adapt to mental or physical impairment. If an impairment is physical, cognitive activity may provide life's most enjoyable activities. The mind can change and specialize in regions. Persons with sight problems may find their hearing enhanced. These kinds of internal modifications probably are happening far more often than we know. If something goes awry in one area, as often happens, pick up and work harder in other areas. Our abilities probably are rarely exhausted, so keep pushing the edge of your ability to grow.

Lifetime Habits

Now that humanity's lifespan is increasing dramatically, it becomes even more important to build habits of cognitive and physical fitness. Cognitive routines probably are much more likely to remain lifetime habits. Our personal reading habits stay very strong, although different from each other. Research for this book took us far away from our usual practices, reinforcing skills developed in graduate schools. Our physical fitness is still evolving and has become part of our daily routines, although reading occupies far more time than does physical fitness. Fitness routines follow our passion for things that require clear thinking and mobility.

Along the life pathway, brain injuries can occur, strokes happen, or other disasters impede full functioning. So far, our wounds have been with bones and heart, each setting back the physical fitness routines. And heart surgery probably set back brain functioning for a while. The prevailing wisdom is to get back into active operation quickly for bone and heart recovery, which is why rehabilitation is required. Our experiences with such problems suggest that the formal repair covered by insurance is a bare minimum of what is needed to regain complete recovery.

An active lifestyle and habits of improving performance are most notable for preventing problems and obtaining a full recovery. All attributes of an active ager are called into play when disasters strike. Those accustomed to training routinely have accumulated the mental, emotional, and muscular discipline and habits required for a rebound from or mitigating the effects of injury and other failures of our body systems. The brain that has trained for fitness has cognitive reserves that can be called into play when needed. The mind that has learned to learn and grow can use the same plasticity to reorganize in ways that compensate for losses in other areas.

Investing for Life

Planning early, training early, and developing active pursuits is for the body what a savings and investment plan is for the financing of a long and active retirement. You are building the reserves for when they are needed in the future, while enjoying the present in the most fruitful, enjoyable, and productive ways. Focusing and spending time on what is important is your most precious asset. Used wisely, it pays great dividends.

Preparing early, long, and consistently is a winner for pleasure today and also solid gold needed for reserves, breakdowns, and accidents likely in the future.

We believe our successful recoveries from surgeries were, in large part, related to our practice and belief that active aging is possible and that many of the behaviors written about here make that possible. Our many investments in education and experiences contribute significantly to the range of choices we have had and the pursuits we still enjoy. If we were pessimistic or believed that older age is mostly about decline, it's doubtful we would even be alive.

If you resign yourself to the thought that "I am just getting old," you already are old and in decline. Focus on being fully active physically and mentally today and every day, and you are living the good life available to most of us who believe it is possible.

Things to Remember

Nothing dulls the mind like endless hours watching mind-numbing TV shows. So many things can be exciting and serve as challenges to imagine and think about. Watching clouds with their endless variations or looking closely at a new blossom can engage thinking. If the outdoors isn't available, watch slow-motion photography of life in the wild, such as a flower blooming, a bee feeding off a flower, or a bat retrieving nectar from a one-night-a-year blossoming saguaro flower. There is much to calm the mind and bring beauty into our lives.

Many facts we learn in college have a half-life of years, rarely remaining with us for decades, and seldom forever. The admonition to become a lifelong learner is good advice.

- Keep up to date on subjects of interest.
- Read about developments in your field of expertise or interest.
- Look for opportunities in your travels for conferences, workshops, and other learning opportunities.

Knowledge is theory populated by facts. Over time, it is not unusual for new artifacts or methods to emerge that render old ideas or opinions obsolete.

Now is the time to try out for new roles in life. We all have skills in some things that, if we worked at them, we could improve. Life presents many opportunities to grow and develop. Early on, Monty built upon his writing talents to begin creating much poetry. And just walking in the neighborhood often yielded an impressive piece of wood to clean, shape a bit, and use as an art object. Add that to a clay class, and that to painting, and now to a new occupation as a painter.

Want to grow in the new line of work and pleasure? Dig in, expand your knowledge, enjoy it, and get better at doing the new thing.

- Want to write another book, dust off old skills, refresh your knowledge of the fields of interest? Try out new theories.
- Design your new life as an older person while opening your worldview and becoming an intellectually stronger person.

Travel was something we did for work, but we still relished learning and just relaxing. As spirituality became a more active part of our lives, a trip to Israel offered many new insights about ancient and current forms of worship. Creating art made travel to Florence and its treasures a memorable trip. Travel companies provide every kind of trip. The local Y, senior center, churches, and a host of other organizations sponsor far more opportunities than one can imagine. Take advantage of these opportunities. A brain that is engaged and growing is likely to remain active and useful throughout life. That is especially true for the most active members of society.

As we age, our passion for things may shift. However, whatever the object of our affection and interest, it is essential to be as positive in your thinking as possible. Repeatedly focusing on negative thoughts can lead to depression, while focusing more on positive thoughts leads in the opposite direction. If your disposition tends to the negative, work on making it more positive. If it is positive, make it more so.

The adage to "fake it until you make it" applies here. "It is going to be a good day" is so much better a way to begin the day than, "I fear this will be a bummer!"

In all of these adventures, keep your loved ones close, your skills and learning on a positive course, and your focus on making each day extraordinary. A lifetime of special days is a blessing. All of life is a journey, so each day is the best of days.

In summary, keeping the brain growing and functioning requires being active. There are many ways to do that, and thinking about and having a life plan to continue to be productive is a core component of that plan. The good life is always a work in progress. It is a learning growth and learning journey. It is necessary to be optimistic about living fully, growing, seeking out ways to improve your performance, and learning new things. These are critical features of the active ager.

CHAPTER FOUR (Q&A)

1. **"Intellect," "intellectual," and similar words conjure up many expressions dealing with brain functioning, such as deep thinking about particular subjects. Sometimes they refer to a specific kind of person who engages in thinking, research, and teaching or speaking out on public issues. How do you mean those words here?**

    Intellectual and cognitive activity dealing with brain function is front and center in North American today because of the increases in Alzheimer's disease, Parkinson's disease, and strokes. This chapter argues strongly for active agers to use their brains in as many ways as they can imagine. Do creative things, solve problems, sleep expecting the mind to bring new ideas to light for you. Please keep it going. Our personal goals, including this book, stemmed, in part, from a strong sense that this is the way to maintain a healthy mental state as long as we live.

    As active agers, one of our primary concerns is to do what is necessary to keep our minds healthy so that our thoughts remain active and in good order. A significant problem for many elderly people is the onset of dementia, which robs them of their thinking abilities, memories, and the motor controls of the mind over bodily functions. In this book, we focus on the kinds of fitness and eating habits that make for proper brain functioning. We also elaborate on how one's learning and thinking can enhance life and keep one's brain in good working order.

2. **So this is about a healthy brain more than some kind of ideal mental ability?**

For us, it is about both a healthy brain and strong mental ability. With a healthy brain, one's mind remains intact and can roam widely over a lifetime of experiences. Brain damage or deterioration can leave one with so little mental ability that daily functioning is hampered. Keep it healthy and use it to promote active aging. And many of the things we do to exercise the body via strength training and aerobics all improve brain function. Good sleep improves brain function. A well-balanced diet can improve brain function.

We are not against improving on our mental abilities and capacities. And we believe that this is possible at all ages. So, attempts to improve and learn are welcomed and likely outcomes for those who live actively.

There is more that can be done to improve mental health. Our thinking capacity is a key to active aging. We can mentally model behavior. We can read, write, plan, direct our actions, and find ways to change our habits. The ability to read these words and consider their ramifications for our own action is very much an intellectual effort. It is something precious and needed throughout life. So keeping one's brain active, engaged with life, and healthy is a very high priority for thinking people.

3. **Have any issues grown in importance for you in this area since chronicling this progress report?**

Few areas of study offer more to research and consider than the brain/mind issues. There's a constant flow of philosophers, mystics, scientists, and religions leaders all speaking out on some aspect of the mind. Reading their beliefs, theories, and research provides ongoing and most interesting engagement. It is not an area of study for those seeking quick answers. Some use compounds for treating diseases while others may use the same compound or its plant origin to elect religious experiences. Both medical and religious uses continue even as those compounds and plants are banned. The same compounds may be used to facilitate and induce creative endeavors while others use them to prepare people for death from cancer.

Our interest in religion, health care, and consciousness puts us in the crossroads of these discussions, so reading and debating the merits of the debates continues. As the printing of this book closes one stage of learning, ideas and issues are rising for new efforts to understand the working of the universe. Are we one with All or separate actors on one stage for a mortal journey, destined for another journey after this? Or is just a phase or part of a single process, or perhaps something not yet imagined? The mind is where we spend most of our time. And the best of that time is when we sense the interconnected of All.

4. Which writings are most important for this chapter?

When it comes to intellectual health, hardly any author can be left out. The physicians often point to the biological aspects of brain and mind. Bredesent deals with the many factors which might cause Dementia and how to deal with them. Even today's political pundits when writing more on societal issues discuss issues of intellectual functioning. Burnett and Evans as well as our chapter on methods deal with important ways of thinking about problems and using mental tools to conceive of and execute plans. One of Monty's courses was titled strategic thinking, pointing more to the mental modeling and ways of thinking that can be useful to managers. Csikszentmihalyi delves deeply into thinking at the cutting edge of knowledge. So read the authors dealing with subjects of interest and you will by doing so engage in an intellectual health activity.

CHAPTER FIVE

Psychology and Aging: It's All In Your Head

Be open to life in the present
Accept yourself, help someone
Live fully, be positive
Talent is for use, not idleness

Want a lift? Go out and play
Enjoy a glass of wine or water
Stretch to reach your goals
Plan ahead, act daily

Meditate for quiet and focus
Show up and be kind
Or just be quiet and enjoy the silence

How can we best describe the aging personality?

Traits, attributes, and stereotypes abound to describe the aging person-ality; there are dozens of analogies, each adding insight. Some see aging as a battle. For others, it's more like an animal or plant; it springs from a seed, grows, matures, propagates, grows older, and dies. Some living things grow to become food for other living things. All living things pass on their characteristics to other living beings. Things, Being, Life comes in so many forms. One's environment shapes much of what we become. The term from "dust to dust" is not inappropriate. Nor is the idea of eternal life for the soul.

For humans, animals, and plants, the genetic lines go on and on. Not every life reproduces, but most do. In fact, in our time, the planet seems to be getting crowded, as more humans manage to reproduce in sufficient numbers to overburden many parts of the land. Over time, we each become a recognizable person, a personality all our very own. Sunny, morose; active, passive; introvert, extrovert; and all of this goes into the aging personality.

Whatever analogy one wishes to use, we humans have a wide vari-ety of personalities, as is the case with body types and mental abilities as well. Families experience variation within their own members among the gene types and the expression of genes. So, whatever metaphor or analogy one uses to describe the human condition, there are many ways and methods for achieving a successful active aging life. As a result, the analogies that fit our lives are many. Learning machines, pacemakers, servants, stewards of gifts, and many others apply. In so many ways, we are adapted to learning how best to live in changing environments. For us, part of this learning comes from our broad exposure from travel to and study of health systems in other countries and consulting with hospitals and other groups throughout the United States.

Barbara studied nursing and hospital administration and prac-ticed those professions in a variety of settings. Monty's college studies led to his being invited to speak with and before hospital audiences at national, regional, and statewide meetings before he worked full time in the health field or studied health administration. Exposure to many types of organizations offered a variety of insights into how to do things. It was from these early exposures to comparative methods and issues that each of us gained our more in-depth insight into how to deal in creative ways with issues of health status and service.

Growing old can be challenging physically and mentally. We exercise to keep the mind and body working. We eat to fuel up for work and life. We build reserves to use in hard times, and those reserves include the challenges that build resilience in our minds. Our travels to Canada offered insights into how to organize for optimizing health status. In England, we learned ways for institutions to deal with problems of aging. Comparative exposure to a variety of ideas was a hallmark for studying issues and seeking the more useful ways to define the questions and to find creative ways of living actively, even when confined to institutional care and services.

Given our time spent in schools, learning, storing knowledge, and exercising our minds, the war we were gearing up to fight was one where the mental challenges could be decisive. Combining formal education in schools with comparative exposure to many institutional solutions gave us an unparalleled opportunity to excel in our field of practice and our daily lives. Given our only modest physical fitness, we didn't anticipate fighting a war of strength and endurance . . . unless the war was one requiring cognitive fitness.

Given the challenges one faces in life, the ones that seem ubiquitous to us are mental. Learning to learn is one of the most basic of skills to master for an active life. Why? Life throws curve balls, and those who can handle them mentally are often the best positioned to prepare for the resources needed to win such battles. Moreover, the actions required are not so much fending off others as fending off the urge to quit working harder or to give up too soon, and to forgo savings for pleasures at the moment. It is the psychological traits that keep one going that matter the most. We spent many years in schools learning, and more doing research and writing. However, formal education isn't the only route to mental toughness and to success in mastering the hurdles one faces over a lifetime.

Can we hold this life together as our sight dims, hearing weakens, and limbs stiffen? Do we have the stamina to adapt to a new environment in a continuing care community in a new state with new people and all kinds of adjustments in freedom and human interactions? The answer is that we do have what it takes to give it a good effort. How do we know this? We have made many moves successfully in the past. We have worked through all kinds of problems. We have faced illness and seen death, not for ourselves yet but for loved ones. Much of what life presents we have managed. When we have sensed weakness in our approach and abilities, we have moved to correct the situations. More schooling, more savings, more dieting, more of whatever is needed to prepare for the contingencies we can anticipate needing.

What holds us together in this new dimension of life? A short answer is our trust in a higher being and our self-confidence.

We have worked hard to develop the habit of mindfulness so we can stay in the moment and respond appropriately to challenges before us. New experiences bombard us daily, and old patterns we have relied on for security now are challenged. Friends die suddenly, and finding our way in a crowded city is taxing. One of us no longer drives a car, so we scramble to see if we should use the limousine service here instead of facing city traffic and aggressive drivers. For every loss we have suffered so far, there has been an alternative approach. That will end someday, but the test for the active ager is to find options as losses occur. When our wakeful awareness dims, so too will life, as we know it slows for its inevitable ending. Our goal is to stay as active as possible throughout, knowing that an end does come. Why be active? Giving in to pain and decline will come soon enough without welcoming it prematurely.

We pride ourselves on being good at problem-solving. For the past year, we worked out new rhythms for shopping and getting our supply of needed medicine and other essentials in a more organized fashion. Fortunately, we live near first-class grocery stores, pharmacies, health care providers, and other services.

At the same time as we are trying to solve immediate problems, we have the urge to be helpful to new people moving into our residential community and asking for reassurance, answers to questions, and companionship, just as we did when we moved in. Meeting life challenges as we go along offers insights into needs likely to arise in the future. Being alert to these needs represents an opportunity to grow in compassion and to prepare for those likely future trends coming to us.

Frequent Challenges Strengthen Our Reserves

Another analogy of aging is us as computers with infinite storage capacity. We keep adding to our memories to augment the mind's ability to access all that we have stored for reasonable solutions. Unlike most modern computers, however, we are ones that write and re-write their programs. Moreover, our capacity seems endless, although like a computer which has flooded out, if we lose our minds, we are without a precious resource for independent living.

Many challenges appear as we decide how to divide our time between scheduled events and quiet moments in our apartment. We ponder when to speak up about uneven service and when to be more patient until we have additional information about a problem. As we look to the future, we wonder how to handle fears of falling and breaking a leg or hip and being moved out of familiar surroundings to a rehabilitation facility focused solely on encouraging people to move and get better. The preparation for war and the walking wounded who leave scarred forever come to mind as we see the ravages of aging in others. However, there remain many for whom suffering in life's battles leaves them lame but their will to stay active remains strong.

Living in a continuing care retirement community (CCRC), we have many supports to cope with the ravages of decline. We have a courteous, respectful staff and attentive neighbors, who make it easy to embrace new realities quickly and positively. Our challenge now is to navigate our current world. Our questions include:

- Do the appropriate responses in our psychic core kick in and provide the right balance and strength as we walk new paths of self-discovery?
- Can a robust psychological skillset help us in our ongoing aging quest?
- Where do we find answers to these questions?

Familiar Territory

Unlike computers, we have written and overwritten our programs many times. Also, we have gone for formal education and experience in fields germane to our main interest—robust good health and high energy. Thus, we are well prepared for finding useful answers in our personal lives, in part because in our professional lives we're dealing with the knowledge about good health and well-being. Those steeped in the culture of other fields need much of the health care knowledge to navigate their personal lives. For many, coming into a CCRC is a new experience. For us, it is more moving into a model that we helped to design and build. Now, of course, with our aging eyes, we can see some of the needs we failed to see in our earlier years. For example, Barbara has excellent teachers who drilled her in grammer; Monty's less well prepared grade school left his with fewer tools of grammar ready for use. Early deficits can linger and hinder one's full flowering of the mind. Hindsight is excellent but rarely useful. All those years of study and a comparative visits to institutions, nations, and cultures now are a valuable adjunct to our search for the best ways to age actively.

Besides probing within our personal experience for this book, we studied many authors writing about their research on human performance. No doubt most of their fundamental ideas about self-fulfillment, high performance, showing respect and love to others, and focusing on the immediate in our environment is helpful. Just by studying many different fields of scholarship and research, we have developed mental reserves capacity, which helps carry us in this new environment.

The Desire for Self-Actualization

Each of us consistently strives for self-actualization. In all of the many life experiences we have had the privilege to encounter, we have sought the appropriate environment where we could be nourished physically, mentally, and also morally. In all of our encounters, we have striven to bloom as a well-developed, secure, loving individuals. Not every attempt is equally successful, but even failure can teach suitable lessons.

Monty has worked at and mastered the roles of husband, father, friend and counselor, writer, explorer, artist, and philosopher. Barbara has striven to be a loving and attentive religious woman, nurse, wife, administrator, teacher, counselor, writer, explorer, and friend. For us, service to others and stewardship of resources to extend that service is a guiding principle in our lives. Since needs seem omnipresent and perpetual, so too does our need to strive to remain active. Without the ability to stay active, life purposes are difficult to fulfill.

Gifts of the Sonoran Desert Years

We cannot discount the intense training we received in stillness, beauty appreciation, and sensitivity to the mysterious and the uniqueness of living with a variety of animals. Our twenty years of retirement in the Sonoran Desert in Tucson, Arizona, offered many insights into fitness, spirituality, the arts, and the challenges of networking and volunteering. Of our many pursuits over the years, creativity and spirituality seem the most inner-directed. However, coming into contact with people, and, in this case, the wildness of the Sonoran Desert have been gifts of great value. Not only were we blessed by the lessons for us in this beautiful natural area but we also had the opportunity to touch the lives of others. For those affected by the spirituality of our home and its arts, the load of life lifted; when someone was attracted to a painting, they connected to a world of beauty and meaning. Both touch the lives of others in a deep and meaningful way. We were blessed living there and, in turn, were able to enrich the lives of others during their visits.

Now that we no longer have the privilege of living in the desert, we are beginning to fully appreciate what a gift we were given in our individual growth to experience the magnificence of continually acting and reacting within the different phases of desert life. We awakened with the sun and went to sleep with its beautiful settings. We studied and became proficient in learning the dangers and gifts of the multitude of animal creatures that shared the habitat with us. Getting in touch with nature's rhythms brought us close to a realization of the quality of life we were living as well. It has a rhythm, a movement. Life comes and goes, but Life never really ends; it merely recycles matter and energy. We are lucky to have had this exposure to nature. Otherwise, in our more narrow human interactions, we might well have missed the larger picture of which we were and continue to be a contributing part.

We were privileged to have extraordinary dogs and cats as part of our family. Their love for us and the gentle ways they guarded and taught us now aches in our souls because they are no longer here with us in our new residence. That too is life; the cycles of different life forms vary from ours. Our lives are short compared with the Saguaro, which lives for 250 to 350 years. We lived among those large plants, and after they died as plants, we used their hardened trunks to create yard art, giving them a resurrected life. The skeletons of those now "dead" giants now grace the territory of our living room. Also, their beauty implanted indelible marks on our psyche and accounted for our tendency to look for beauty everywhere, to respect all earthly creatures, and to honor the magnificence of the universe.

Because of our Sonoran experience, Monty is now a full-fledged artist, Barbara is more quiet and introspective, and both of us strive for more profound creativity and psychological depth. Our desert experience deepened our self-confidence and increased our desire to live each day to the fullest. Our passion for Active Aging became our mantra in the Sonoran Desert.

Other Learnings

Now in our late-eighties (Yipes!), we are learning other lessons. We are nearing the end point of our aging life and mixing with others our age each day. We are continually aware that as people become older, more infirm, and more dependent on others, living can be quite a challenge. Older people generally seek environments where nourishing food and drink will be available, where they will be safe from the vagaries of environmental hazards, criminals, and others who would bring them harm. They seek environments where they can safely visit with friends and engage in group activities and support one another in reaching their particular goals of self-actualization.

During our two years in Kansas City, we have learned that these environments desired by older people take many forms, such as friendly neighborhoods with children and other loved ones nearby. Others may need and benefit from a community that offers supportive services and a rich assortment of social programs and inclusive living environments.

Some people stay in their homes, some move in and share living quarters with other older adults, and some accept the help of governments, churches, and voluntary organizations that provide elderly housing assistance.

Finally, some seniors search desperately for basic needs and safety and roam the cities looking for homeless shelters, quiet parks, and sometimes-safe jails to get by day to day. In these cases, self-actualization is a much lower priority than daily survival. For many, even the most basic needs are difficult to secure.

Wisdom of Aging

Looking at life now from the vantage point of eighty-five-plus years plus behind us, we are beginning to exhibit wisdom about where we are in the life cycle. This new understanding helps us to more honest in our acceptance of ourselves.

From this perspective, we seem to be more open to expressing our true feelings about relationships, the state of the world, and our retirement community environment. We are striving to be positive in our stance toward our immediate environment and toward our chaotic world.

Living in the Present

Another part of our newly found wisdom is the acknowledgment of the sense of living fully in the present moment. We know this current time is all we have. Therefore, we don't dwell on past tragedies or mistakes we have made. We try to focus our energy on what is happening now and strive to be the best we can be. Being present is Active Aging at its best!

Over the years, both of us have worked at living in the present. To convert this idea into the process of Active Aging, we strive to be open to the aging process and the resultant life adjustments this reality presents.

Because we have lived extraordinary lives, both individually and as a couple, we have acquired valuable experience in accepting and dealing positively with our feelings of fear, discouragement, love, or irritation. We work at living in the present and not obsessing over past mistakes and worries. We continually strive to confront and deal positively with life situations that occur right here, right now.

Acceptance of Weaknesses

In our everyday life, we no longer sugarcoat the realities of diminished balance and hearing. We can seek assistance when walking or moving around in unfamiliar areas. We also respect and thank younger people who patiently give us directions when we appear baffled in a new situation. We have discovered that today's society knows and accepts the fact that we have lost stamina and coping skills that were fully present in earlier times.

It's okay. We seek help when we need it and show gratitude to those who help us. We learn here in the retirement community that this is the reality we present today. We will seek help when we need it and are grateful to those who assist us. We no longer aspire to complete independence. We live in a world of specialization and at a time when our specialty knowledge half-life is short. We are dependent on others, recognize this, and seek ways to cover our needs in times of stress. Times of need occur and will come more often with advanced age.

We are also striving for positive life goals. To this end, we strive to be positive and loving in our daily interactions with each other and all of our fellow residents and our remaining relatives.

Looking back at the past two years, we realize the major lifestyle transformation we have accomplished. One day we were free as birds at our desert oasis. The next day Monty was faced with open heart surgery, and our idyllic world turned upside down. Coping in the desert was no longer an option; we needed to move on.

To facilitate Monty's optimal recovery, we chose to move to Kansas City to be near cardiology specialists we had previously worked with as health care consultants. The regular rhythms of living in our desert neighborhood, being in constant touch with friends, and familiar routines were disrupted. Loved ones offered support, but they were limited in what they could do during this lifestyle change.

We had long decided that our next move should be to a place where most of our needs and wants could be found within walking distance or a short ride away. Our new environment places us within walking distance of medical resources and minutes away from many of the most important cultural features of Kansas City. We are in the heart of the city, at least compared to our desert retreat, which was fifteen miles out, adjacent to a wilderness area.

Our move to Kansas City required major downsizing; we reduced our living space by 80 percent and gave up acres of land for enjoying. The loss of highly visible night skies and connection to nature are significant losses. Many changes facing older persons require reshuffling resources, disruptions in long-held friendships, and the shock of starting life in an entirely different environment.

We sought this change with the idea that it would be a refreshing way to begin the last leg of our life journey. As we write this, we are passing through the 85-year-old range, which signals "Old Old" age. Yes, for these years, although we are less physically able and energetic than we once were, we are amid the abundant cultural resources of a great city. We are again in a learning environment. We pursue our interests, listen to great music, attend lectures, and concerts. We do many things with ease because our immediate environment offers such riches. Our sense of the need for more learning is at work. We live actively here.

All of us yearn to be positively engaged in life and psychologically whole when encountering the challenges of living in today's complex society. It is critical for us, as mature human beings, to be skilled in mastering today's sophisticated culture. We cannot hide behind the notion that twenty years ago everything was more straightforward and thus say," I want to go back to that time!" No, that is not a reality for us. The way forward is to seek challenge, not to pull back from it. The road ahead is to meet the challenges and enjoy the encounters. We learn and grow from the difficulties. It is the direction of our lives.

Acceptance of a Complex Environment

To get geared up for this battle with our current reality, we seek psychological grounding that reinforces the idea that we have to be patient with ourselves and remember each of us is a person who has good and bad qualities and is striving to grow positively.

We need to develop sensing mechanisms that help us better understand the world we live in now. Developing skill in this realm, we need to listen to and understand the daily news, engage in discussions with others about current events, and take well-thought-out positions on critical issues. Being aware of the complexity of the environment and adapting to it is a crucial variable in being a successful active ager.

A rule of thumb in this regard is to go with what life presents in the here and now, study the critical variable in each complicated situation, and take a stand within yourself about where you are in this societal give and take.

Our experience suggests that this is a positive approach to dealing with sticky societal situations. Of course, if the implications of this solution mean loss of work, or illness, or other adverse events, instead of Happy Day, the message might be, "Here we go again, another challenge. What can I do today to move out of this hole?" Alternatively, for some, no doubt, the message is simply HELP!

The bottom line in this discussion is that the positive Active Ager should spend a considerable amount of time defining personal goals that are positive and other-directed. Also, one needs to embrace life events one minute at a time while responding positively to the majority of life situations along with their complexity.

Accept the Flow, Focus on the Present

The complexity of living in today's world is not going away. We want to be a part of it while at the same time harnessing our positive energy to lead a wholesome existence.

A plethora of literature today focuses on living in the moment, not being distracted by the ebb and flow of meaningless chatter and irrelevant events. It behooves us to spend more time understanding the ideas of Mihaly Csikszentmihalyi, the noted psychologist who developed the notion of flow; i.e., focusing on the task at hand while harnessing all of your energy to accomplish what is before you.

Several years ago, we had the good fortune to go on a walking tour of Switzerland led by Mihaly Csikszentmihalyi, who was then a University of Chicago professor and author of *Flow*. We hiked the mountains in the Swiss Alps during the day, and in the evening, we discussed with Mihaly his research and emerging ideas about flow.

How exciting it was to hear him talk about this concept of experiencing the human-world intersection. He reminded us that some professionals such as surgeons, artists, athletes, musicians, and chess players become so involved in activities they love that nothing else matters to them. As a result, they are ready to invest more attention to the process involved in the project without worrying about an immediate return.

Some people argue that the flow state favors the young, the artist, or a person training for a critical mission or technical procedure. So we ask, can flow apply to people who are aging? Our experience suggests yes, that flow is a state of being that can become real for active people who are still growing and still striving to excel in some way.

One can argue persuasively that the flow state could be a long-term goal for anyone on the aging path. People who are getting older have much more time and space for things other than work activities. How do you fill in this space? Our professional lives and skillsets have morphed into this case study on active aging and areas as conducive to flow as ever.

Those who are growing older and not afraid to try new things branch out in creative endeavors. Watching Monty transition from a high-powered consultant, writer, and executive to a painter has been a critical case study in moving into the flow state.

He began slowly in Tucson with found objects converted to art pieces. He took a few classes in ceramics, one in painting with acrylics, and then he liberally decorated our home at Spirit Base Camp and our four-plus-acre property. He spent hours in his makeshift studio in the garage, mixing colors, constructing masks, and making small figurines that we gave to friends and visitors.

Just as he was arranging to show some of his art at a shop, heart surgery intervened. He did sell a few pieces, but the real reward for painting was becoming hooked on an open-ended new career as an artist! Monty spent much of his time in a flow state. The art enriched his life and those of others around him.

Barbara also achieved a flow state in her own way; she accepted a request by the CCRC administration to work with other residents to start a Friendly Neighbors Program (FNP). This FNP proved to be an exciting new adventure for her and a blessing for the residents who now got visits when moved about among the many treatments and housing modalities.

Here at Bishop Spencer Place, we have art classes that result in beautiful pieces created by many residents. Our life enrichment coordinator commented that residents with dementia do some of the most precise work. These individuals connect deeply with their work and develop intricate designs and blend beautiful colors.

Strive for Resilience

Aging people encounter many challenges to well-being, including chronic illnesses, periods in acute care and rehabilitation facilities, the death of loved ones, and disruption of working and living arrangements. Resilient people can adjust to these situations more easily than people with more structured lifestyles.

How does one develop this positive trait of resiliency? We think through much hard work and focused attention to dealing with real life in stressful situations. Those who attain success in this area seem to have a strong sense of purpose in their life and current work. They acknowledge the vagaries of their current age, and they work with the resultant physical and mental changes that occur daily. Through the daily grind, people with remarkable resilience manifest a soft sense of humor. They also work hard to develop a creative view of the world, which at times keeps them balanced when everyone else in the room appears deranged.

As we come to know and appreciate more fully our neighbors here at Bishop Spencer Place, we are amazed at a large number of people with noticeable resiliency. People who have undergone knee and hip surgery are up and trying to walk the halls the first day after surgery. These residents will tell you that they are not going to let surgery get them down. They will do everything they are told to do in order to return their quarters and resume the projects they are involved in.

By contrast, people who resist change are rigid in their thinking about how the world should revolve around them, and they lack a sense of humor. They refuse to endure the discipline of physical therapy, expect to be given extra attention for everything they request, and do not tolerate the usual aches and pains of post-surgery rehabilitation. Life fails to reward such personal neglect and often leaves these people less able than they might have been had they done the rehab in a more persevering manner.

Positive Portrait

So how should an Active Ager manifest psychological health? Some of their characteristics include the following:

- They know who they are and focus on becoming a better human being, aware of their good and bad qualities.
- They experience little stress because they are open to surprises and change that come unexpectedly.
- When confronted with new challenges, they accept whatever presents itself without dictating outcomes.
- They live thoughtfully and confidently while resisting social pressures to behave in a particular way.
- They exude confidence in moving and working in varied environments.
- They are sought out by peers for friendship and support.
- They exhibit a sense of serenity and keen focus as they show people respect, do assigned work, and engage in creative pursuits.
- They cultivate and exhibit a sense of humor in the ups and downs of life.
- They are assertive and skilled in communication with individuals and groups.
- They display confidence in personal and work situations.
- They have an active social life.

**If life seems to slow a bit too much,
perk up and become more active.
Active begets activity. It is self-reinforcing.
It is in our nature to be active and self-
healing. So if you haven't already absorbed
the message, to be active is to be alive.**

Finishing Strong

Now in our tidying-up phase of life, we must heal essential relationships that have frayed. Now we need peace. However, Monty will no doubt have paint on his hands when he passes away and a working manuscript in progress. Barbara may go while trying to help a neighbor in distress.

CHAPTER FIVE (Q&A)

1. Are aspects of personality and individual approaches that have been helpful to you in this active aging life?

There are several. Dealing with problems as they arise is far better than putting them off; delay leaves the problem to fester and become worse. This also applies to setting and meeting one's goals and aspirations. It is helpful on a day-to-day basis to think about one's fitness and eating goals, consider what is ahead for the day, and try to anticipate problems that might arise. It also helps to break grand goals into things that can be done TODAY!

2. If we find ourselves being pessimistic and negative in life situations, should any of the suggestions in this chapter stimulate us to move in different directions?

Yes. Obsessing over the past is wasted energy in the same way as worrying about things that might never happen. If one often thinks of the past, it is almost impossible to not dwell on things one might have done differently to have experienced a better outcome. Of course, one can't ever change the past; it is gone. One way to dispel the fascination of the past and the what-ifs is to forgive yourself for the supposed error or forgive the person whose transgressions might have caused the adverse event or outcome.

Trying to overthink the kinds of negative things that might happen in the future can have adverse effects in the present. Planners, like us, try to imagine the many ways in which the future might unfold. We do that to discover what might be a small service to offer someone in the present to change future outcomes. The aim is to keep the goals for the future in mind in the present moment.

The present is where action can and does happen. We can do the thing needed or not. Do the right thing today, and tomorrow is more likely to be a good day.

Obsessing over the past and possible futures can be very harmful. Both the past and future possibilities can be mined for ideas that can be acted upon in the present. Like many things, how one uses the past recollections and future thinking makes a big difference in the value of such thoughts.

3. **It isn't always easy to stop thinking about mistakes made in the past or pitfalls that might well attend a new direction in one's life. Are there things that help deal with such issues?**

There are many ways in which one can deal with the anxieties associated with past mistakes and future challenges. Much of this book is dedicated to some of those: For instance, physically fit people seem to weather adversity better. People of faith can often call on their faith and fellow members for support. And our comments on social relations are all relevant for this issue as well. Living in the present negates the psychological dilemma of visiting past traumatic experiences that have already been resolved.

There are many other things one might do: Meditation to alleviate stress and anxiety is helpful. Visualization of positive outcomes is useful. Dealing with issues as they come up is helpful. In our tiny household, we lament the small size of our living space from time to time. But cleaning up and putting things back into order is easy and helps to keep that little space available for the next event.

One administrator we know was reputed to never leave a meeting without making sure that someone else was assisgned the responsibility for taking the next action step. That may not be the best way to act, but pinning down responsibility for the next needed act is helpful, whoever is to do the work.

4. Are there other factors that stand out for you?

There is one factor that stands out. Being positive, greeting the world with the expectation of good occurring helps in most situations. Having a general disposition to expect good things to happen makes life less stressful. We are reminded of the story of the room with a large pile of dung. Some see it and turn away, envisioning no good to come of the encounter. But others find it to be a hopeful moment because, as one child said, "With all that horse shit, there must be a pony in here somewhere." Remember the adage, if you draw a lemon, make lemonade.

Monty was once an Armory Officer for a Bomb Wing readying for deployment. One of his tasks was ordering holsters for the 38-caliber pistols for air crew members to use. Just days before the deployment, the holsters arrived, with a strap to hold the gun in place. The strap was too short to cover the gun but long enough if put through the trigger guard. So he simply announced that the holsters had a special feature to keep from accidentally pulling the trigger when the gun was in the holster. The crews accepted this lemonade answer. It was a mistake, the order was a lemon and it did require some fast rebranding. So practice looking for alternatives for things that can and do go awry.

5. Individual personality and actions are considered important considerations for active aging. Who are some of the writers who have most influenced your work?

Some of the most important lessons about how to live one's life comes not from the academic writings and influences but the virtues taught more by family, culture and faith teaching. The value of hard work, the necessity for doing for oneself, and learning new techniques or trades to get ahead came early and often. We knew that we were given much and had an obligation to develop out tralents and use them to improve ourselves and those around us.

In schools there were many teachers. In graduate studies academics in many disciplines shared their knowledge and methods so that we could think about problems and issues we face in our lives, and especially, in the workplaces we studied. Maslow, Rogers, Kabot-Zinn, Pinker, Kornfield, Ryff, Csikszentmihalyi, and dozens of physicians-scientist who note psychological factors which influence health, all influenced our thinking along the way. Which ones the most is difficult to discern. It is also difficult to impossible to remember the sequence in which some of the ideas we ultimately espouse were acquired. It difficult to ascertain whether an author taught us something or something they said or for which our mind found another meaning. For example, Richard Blau and one of his student, Richard Scott did a study and noted the use of posting results for all to see and using that as a control device. Feedback was what I recall taking away as the meaning their finding. Later I discussed my take away and the authors intentions with Prof. Scott and he said, I don't recall that we had any intention of saying what you took away from that chart. I can freely acknowledge the takeaway I had, but unknown or unintended by the authors. No doubt the mixing and matching of ideas results in creative thinking. This is likely many ideas in this book that build on the encounters with other minds. That is the nature of communication among humans. In our consulting work we always consider the outcomes to be joint products, stemming in large part from the interaction of minds and thoughts of many. This book is loaded with the mental products of many minds. What you see is but the latest iteration coming from our current understanding of how things work.

CHAPTER SIX

Spiritual Wellness: A Greater Purpose

Religion pathways vary
Individuals choose
Spirituality beckons
Faith undergirds purpose
Purpose strengthens
our desire to serve

Lead a positive life
Live with love
Serve others
Be kind

Whichever path is taken
Love one another
Show up
Act

Spirituality

Spirituality may be the most challenging active aging component to discuss, yet ultimately one of the most rewarding. Spirituality cuts to the core of who we are and what we hope to become as we relate to a God-anchor in our lives. This idea of God in our lives is a broad concept that takes years to understand and live. It reflects the creature/God interaction in a plethora of religious organizations throughout the world. It also implies that each person connects to someone or something more important than themselves. A person's relationship with God is individual, sacred, and often attached to a church structure and hierarchy.

It is also true for us that our sense of "Spirit"/"God" has changed over the years and is much more individualized as we age. Regardless of our different church affiliations (Barbara's is Catholic and Monty's is Episcopalian), both of us are very aware of a spiritual presence surrounding us and influencing our lives.

Monty is aware of a more significant spiritual and consciousness presence as he produces one original piece of work after another. Some of this sense of existence is that of flow; being there is all there is. It is a bubble of time and has a unique character. The artistic process demands his silence, full attention to the task, and the surrender of his inclinations to a driving force within him to move in a particular direction. The connection to more significant power in his life drives his work.

Barbara's spirituality manifests through her deep molding in prayer and meditation during her time as a consecrated religious woman. The results of this internal process are seen through her striving to be sensitive to the perceived physical, social, psychological, and/or spiritual needs of people. Through her years of meditation and silence, she can quickly pick up and sense the needs of people around her.

Each of us has a different view of religion and spirituality and its reach into the realm of the supernatural worlds. Our faith and belief systems are profoundly individualized and reinforced by our relationship with God. Individually, we do not agree on the various tenets of a particular church, such as Catholic or Baptist or Jewish. However, we come together in accepting the importance of spirituality as separate from a religious sect. We both agree that spirituality motivates us at the deepest levels of our being. It provides the stimulus for us to contribute to our community, culture, and the world.

In another sense, religion disseminates certain doctrines and practices that followers subscribe to and model for others. Spirituality, on the other hand, guides a person to find meaning in their life without having to carry out prescribed practices and rituals. It also becomes a sensing mechanism to find people of like-minded ideas to come together and serve others according to the values and directions of the group the person is living in. At times, the ambiance and direction of the group dictate the behavior of the people who subscribe to the group's articulated values.

Defining Terms
Religion is institutional-based, with religious leaders defining the procedures for their congregations to worship, relate to the church, and carry out church-sponsored activities. Spirituality is something deep within an individual. It is a way of relating to God and loving and accepting this Divine Being as a vital part of life.

As we age, religion and spirituality become even more important realities that we seek to understand and integrate into all of our life decisions. We agree that belief systems are abundant about God, and it is up to us to choose what is right for the integrity of our personhood.

Our desert habitat in Tucson enhanced our learning about growth in spiritual wellness. After living there and experiencing its beauty and ancestor-rich environment, we named our home Spirit Base Camp (SBC). We saw it as an oasis where people could be free to search the realms of the Spirit in their way and at their own pace. In this sacred place, we both grew in grace, wisdom, and understanding of the Spirit. SBC was also a place from which we could travel wide but always return. It was home. In this process, visitors caught the energy and found their sense of the Spirit/God in that sacred space.

Spirit Base Camp energized us about the power of reinforcing our sensitivities to the spiritual side of life. We couldn't study the desert animal kingdom and not be astounded by the interdependency of one species with another in warding off deadly predators, foraging for food, protecting younger species, and heroically facing death when it was time. We grew in the realization that the spiritual side of life drove the life cycle. There was a vital force within the plants, trees, cactus, and desert animals that was the dominant force operating all around us. Over the years, we finally got that lesson and became more dependent on the Spirit as our guiding force.

These new insights do not demean those who dedicate themselves to a particular church and its doctrines. However, as a couple, we have spent most of our energy in developing an active spirituality, which has recently become the guiding force for our life.

This spirituality is a search for meaning and purpose in life. It focuses on personal values that guide our actions, emphasizes that we are the continuum between past and future generations, and reinforces the concept that we connect to a Higher Power. It also stresses the need for a deep interior life of prayer, meditation, and a quiet and continual reflection of one's purpose in life.

In this discussion, we focus more closely on spirituality than on religion, although we recognize the two concepts are interrelated.

However, we believe spirituality has a psychobiological basis that needs cultivation and constant attention. We support the idea that as people grow in spirituality, they come to appreciate what they have in common with the faith traditions of others.

Broadening this distinction further, a religious person accepts a specific set of beliefs as valid and observes a prescribed set of rituals mandated by a particular religious denomination. For example, a person of the Christian religion believes Jesus is God's Son and commemorates baptism and receives communion. A person of the Muslim faith believes Allah is God and is the same God as Abraham's God. The Koran nourishes their observation of Ramadan and other holy days.

Deepening our unique spirituality gives us great freedom to find God in everything we do. We know an active Presence is leading us, helping us respond to people in need, guiding us in deep quiet to find greater meaning in everything that happens. Keeping in touch with this Spirit also gives us the freedom to seek examples of a Prime Mover in Buddhist traditions, Jewish teachings, Protestant and Catholic Church teachings. We are free to find God wherever He manifests. I am open to growing spiritually. We can do so without being stopped by particular church rules or obligations. Spirituality does not require a person to be a member of any church.

As active agers, we are becoming more sensitive to the Spirit working with us and helping us become more fully evolved as loving, compassionate, spiritual beings, while at the same time we support the efforts of local churches working within larger congregations.

So where are we on this journey right now? God is guiding us, speaking to us, and helping us grow more spiritually aware. We sense His presence, loving those close to us more fully and responding quickly to people who may need assistance. At the same time, we are growing in a more profound respect for organized religion and the essential roles that various religious groups play in our society. They stand as symbols of a better way to live life fully and with love. Religion plays a vital part in our family, social, and community life, and we respect this phenomenon.

Personal Musings

Our early individual experiences with religion and spirituality were very different. Barbara became a Christian through immersion learning, having been raised in an Irish Catholic family and then joining and living in a religious order for eighteen years. Monty received subtle messages from his loving family and friends but hardly any formal theological training. However, as he assumed his adult responsibilities as a father, professional executive, writer, and researcher, he grasped and lived the significance of a relationship with a Higher Power. When we both discovered the life-giving strength of Spirit Base Camp, we grew in spiritual agility in building an intense interior life, helping others in need and flexing our creative mental skills. Both stories follow.

Barbara's Spirit Journey

God has always been a strong presence in my life. As a small child, I prayed every night before going to sleep that God would protect us, watch over the world, and solve problems for our family and others. The presence of a Higher Power was always real to me, and I relied on it for guidance. As a young child, I loved the Catholic religious women, called Sisters, who taught me in school. They served God full time. These women had a profound influence on me for the first thirty years of my life. In grade and high school, they helped me understand the core tenets of the Catholic Church; i.e., God as a loving Father, Christ as a Redeemer and Teacher; and the Holy Spirit as a Prime Life Guide.

I also learned the essential elements of prayer, meditation, and keeping attuned to the Spirit as a daily practice. This regular interior work gave me the energy and courage to delve deeper into a dedicated spiritual life. I learned to carry on the work of the Catholic Church by serving others with love and compassion.

My school years at a Catholic high school exposed me to the fantastic skills of our intelligent teachers who served as our faculty. They were models of kindness and prayerfulness to their students and to all the less-fortunate people they ministered to outside of their educational responsibilities. These women, wholly dedicated to God, revealed a pathway for me. I wanted to be like them. After one year of college, I joined a congregation of religious women and had the privilege of living with this outstanding group of women who loved God, the Catholic Church, and all the people they served.

Because of my experience in this unique religious environment, I was able to pursue education to become a nurse and hospital administrator. I served eighteen years of my life in various parts of the country where our religious community had hospitals. Besides developing managerial skills running complex health care organizations, I also grew in prayerfulness and responding to people in physical and spiritual pain. Working to serve the sick and poor can be taxing, making it necessary to ground oneself in daily periods of quiet, meditation, and prayer to prepare for service to people in need.

In the 1960s, the Catholic Church was rethinking its stance to the world. The Second Vatican Council, formed by the church hierarchy, met for months pondering the role of the church in the modern world. Many creative ideas emerged. One of those ideas expanded roles for religious women in the priesthood and church administration. Another idea included easing restrictions on birth control. These were the same issues I was grappling with in my mind.

Sadly, these new ideas were set aside for this particular council by the church leaders. The Vatican Council held much promise, but it was stifled by influential people who did not want, at that time, to move boldly into the future. Being impatient with this rate of change, I decided to try another form of service outside the Catholic Church.

After eighteen years, I left a gifted religious group of women to pursue earthly realms of service. Even though I left this unique environment, I did not cease to grow spiritually, and I continued to serve the needs of others as a Christian woman living in a secular world. At this time in my life, I also was introduced to people of various Christian, Jewish, and Buddhist traditions.

After living in a convent, I found the larger world filled with many individuals with various religious orientations committed to serving others with love and dignity. This diverse group of people was energized with God and committed to making the world around them better. Some were as spiritually advanced as my convent colleagues. As I grew older and more independent, I realized that God, as I knew and loved Him, had always been a strong force in my life and would remain so. However, God was also a strong force in the lives of many outside my church. At this point, growth in spirituality, not just in Catholicism, became a focus in my life.

My perceptions about the world and the multiple ways people worship the Supreme Being, the Prime Mover, or their Buddha became increasingly alive to me. I realize now in my eighties that my primary tasks, as I attempt to grow spiritually, are to confront and accept the loss of loved ones, physical illness, reduced independence, and my mortality. I also know that I will be called upon to help others confront these fundamental issues. Contact with a Supreme Being is an essential support in my life to do this work.

Monty's Spirit Journey

My exposure to religious and spiritual ideals has been different from Barbara's. Under the guidance of my parents, I was taught to be respectful and helpful to my neighbors and friends. Our values were grounded in the principles of Protestant Christian biblical traditions. I was conscientious about honesty in all my dealings with others and contributed to the economic survival of my family by working: At eight of nine years of age, I was earning any spending money. At age fourteen, I drove a laundry truck. And at sixteen, I entered a steady five- to six-days-a-week job in the weave room of a cotton mill. Also, helping neighbors in need was the norm for our family and myself.

There was no emphasis in my family on growing spiritually or being a church-going Bible-Reading Christian. For us, it was about the values of a loving family, doing our share of the daily work, earning to support oneself, being kind to friends and neighbors, and showing honesty and respect to others, which included everyone. Racial segregation was the norm, but showing respect was accorded to all, not by race or gender. We were taught that older people have dignity and deserve respect, and that include all races. There were no nursing homes or retirement places, so families lived together, working and sharing their lives from beginning to end.

My family didn't attend church often, although I remember going a few times. However, God and Jesus were not strangers, they have a presence at our home. Growing up in the South, I knew that there were churches that some people attended regularly. I knew them mostly as Baptist, Presbyterian, Methodist, and others. It was conventional wisdom that God sent his Son Jesus to save us. Salvation was by grace, not something one earned. However, the values that went with it were dominant, and God's word as laid out in the Bible was law. I don't recall ever being encouraged to read the Bible, but it was available in the house as a sure guide to Christian living.

Some of our close relatives lived thirty miles away. Having no car, we didn't visit often. Those we visited were deeply religious. As I left for the Korean War, Aunt Etta gave me a small booklet of biblical quotations that I kept in my wallet; my only Bible lessons were from that little booklet. Some of those quotes became an integral part of my life.

A critical lesson that stuck with me is that God gives us our talents and that God, the Master, expects us to invest and use those talents wisely and multiply them for his later return. We are stewards, not entirely free agents to fritter away the opportunities given. We were sent for a purpose to grow, develop, and serve in the manner of the Golden Rule. In short, use well what is there at birth, and be a servant to others, especially those in need. That became a guide for me, so when I learned that lifelong learning was the gift to me, it grew even more critical over the years. I would find myself wondering, *Who doesn't know that?* Later studies in economics taught many of the same virtues. And readers who have reached this point in the book already know how strongly I/we hold these values.

I also frequently think of the verse where Jesus said—and here I say what I remember, not what current versions of the Bible may record—"Whenever two or more gather in my name, there I am also." That is a strong message—invoke my name as you gather, and you are with me and I with you. Being in the presence of Jesus sounds like paradise to me. He is with us when we are together in sacred space. It is a message of total presence now, not just a presence to be met or seen in an afterlife. But here this speaks of a spiritual presence, not a physical presence. Those who seek a universal consciousness might be looking for and seeing or sensing this kind of existence, or so I often imagine.

Over the years, I have read about and shared ideas with others of different spiritual traditions. For me, it means we are fully alive and filled with meaning, purpose, and potential right now, at this moment. We have a destiny in our hands one day at a time. Yesterday is gone; it has little meaning for today, and we can't change it. Moreover, tomorrow never really comes. But count on tomorrow coming. Act as if you will live forever, and live fully expecting that. In doing so, you will optimize the life you have. So real opportunity is right before us, but only in the day, this day when choices are made and action taken. We can think and work on things in the present.

Now I am fully aware of being part of something much larger and unseen by our normal sensing mechanisms. In my Air Force days, I studied electronics and learned of atoms moving along solid objects unseen but interacting with force over long distances. I learned over the years of physics experiments that have detected particles so small they penetrate mountains without touching or being stopped. In the desert years, I saw the unlimited universe in such a small way while learning of its immense spread to unknown horizons, and disappearing, apparently, into black holes.

I know from long years that my brain/mind is not disconnected from others fields of energy and that thoughts, seemingly local, come during the day and night and illuminate my thinking. In poetry, words flow as if already written. In painting, colors emerge, snuggle in close, and bring their uniqueness to expressions of beauty. I am part of a larger whole, no doubt of that, and interacting in ways unplanned and often sought and productive of good. It is as I believe the Buddhists say: We are Not Two with the universe, although neither are we just one. We are not alone but belong in a deep way. We are not just the Ego. We are Not Two with All.

Our Shared Journey

The teachings of the Christian faith give purpose and meaning to life. The building blocks of the pathways we carve for ourselves build upon that foundation, and our spiritual paths infuse those lessons.

We both know that this gives life in the present a deeper meaning. As we pay attention to what is in front of us, to do the things that enhance our health and bring about needed action and change, we are thus living out our mission to serve. Does this mean not planning for the future? No, what is in front of us right now is a step in the direction of our best ideas of what the future can be for us.

These mental models are always working, finding the immediate actions to move us in the direction of our thoughts and models for the future. To us, spiritual life is a life lived fully in the present. We are from dust, and to dust, from matter to matter, we shall return. To us, living a spiritual life honors the realities of life as it is given. Living a life of stewardship and service is a spiritually satisfying life. It is a life lived fully, now, as we have it. Now, when we have it. It can have purpose and meaning if fully lived in the present.

For Monty, awareness of being in a universe of connections and presence is most strongly felt when writing or painting, when engrossed in a creative project. For him, when the mind is stilled, time flows swiftly as new things emerge. More so as he engages in creative projects. He serves others by helping them solve problems.

For Barbara, prayer and meditation is a daily practice. Her days are filled helping people, being present for them, trying to stay in the "now." She is in service as a life mandate. Finding God in stillness and life circumstances is also a principal goal for her.

We continuously mentally model possible futures, and we imagine many ways to solve problems. Human reasoning came to us via the Greeks with Aristotle and Plato modeling it for us. We as humans have marvelous brains that can remember and perhaps draw lessons from reading about the past of many throughout history. Moreover, our spirituality says, "Pay attention to what is before you, act on it, use your talents in service. Take care; be wise." Of course, that is an aspiration, one that animates our lives. It has become our accepted way of living.

This type of thinking is the bedrock for us. We never knowingly pass up opportunities to improve on the "talents" given to us. Have we made mistakes? Of course, and we deeply regret them. Although we believe it is best to let go of attachment to outcomes: however, the instances of unkindness stick the longest.

Coming from different religious backgrounds, we have different approaches to honoring God. However, we both believe that our role in life is stewardship—using what our best gifts express. Life is a living process, lived a day at a time. We have our lodestar—faith in the power of the moment. The now, our consciousness, makes it possible to be alert to what is before us at the moment. Our lodestar is a faith that while we are here and present, we are not alone and life has meaning. Purpose in life isn't from somewhere else or some other source. The use of life is within our being to discern and the actions needed to serve that purpose. In many ways, we are masters of our fate. In even more profound ways, we are created to live out the life given to us. We are part of what is. Moreover, what is exists at the moment.

Spirit Base Camp Journey

After many years of exciting, stressful, and demanding professional work as teachers, researchers, and consultants, we founded and named Spirit Base Camp (SBC) in Tucson. We intended to find a new path for this phase of our lives, to rebuild our fitness and enhance the spiritual side of living. SBC, a place of Spirit, a spiritual retreat, a place to commune with God, the Universe, and the Spirits. Our retirement home was the place of coming together, growing again. We were not mere owners or tenants but stewards. Our gift was to have this natural treasure be a gift to others as well. Mindful of the need to be connected to others, we also sought a neighborhood where we could live more in community.

Spirit Base Camp taught us that in order to give life meaning, our responsibility is to discern how best to build our retired life in changed circumstances. We must again design a life pathway. Building on the past, energy goes to opportunities and ways to serve.

To live fully in the present is to be in a continuous mode of building and rebuilding a life.

The time spent at SBC was very much a spiritual journey. We named our home Spirit Base Camp invoking the idea of being with God, the Spirit and the All. Being there itself was a form of affirmation of living in paradise. Assuming we are created to be purposeful and fruitful, as religions seem to say, then what was our purpose in finding this place near a wilderness area? Night skies there are as dark as one could get near any city in the nation. We found the ideal place to experience a connection to the greater life of the Universe. We were home, our new base camp. We had freedom to explore the Spirit World.

The purpose-driven life doesn't end with each chapter. It goes on and evolves.

At SBC, our goal was to find how best to serve as stewards of the gifts we'd been given. Monty's journey manifested itself in explorations in the arts. For Barbara, it was reaching out to others in service. She formed a Neighborhood Watch, and she went to the University of Arizona to retrain to become a hospice nurse. She also found new creative outlets in gourmet cooking, house decorating, and entertaining. As we became more skilled in being attentive to the Spirit, we became more attuned to the needs of others. After 9/11, both of us became rededicated to our country by helping organize a Medical Reserve Corps Unit and helping public officials recruit volunteers for emergency preparedness. We had the requisite skills and knowledge to do the job; as stewards of what we have, it fell to us to use them for the betterment of the community. That represents our beliefs as much as many other things. We are here; we build upon what we have and use it in the best ways possible to serve the community.

We also discovered in observing the wildlife that surrounded our home that living in the moment was the norm. We began to explore this maxim in depth. Become mindful, do one thing at a time, and concentrate fully on the task at hand. These lessons became guides, embedded beliefs. In everything, we tried to find the Spirit at work. This search for deeper meaning exemplifies our approach to life now.

> **Our belief is that if we should live to one hundred, it is essential that we live each day fully, staying active, moving forward, not sitting back and becoming mere observers.**

We do not seek to live to one hundred but realize it is up to us to prepare as if we might. Today, for instance, instead of deciding to get some supplies for an existing art form, a drawing tablet for a new art project became an interesting project, another journey on the adventure we call living until we stop.

Living in the present has become a powerful way to stabilize our lives and become more spiritual. Solving problems when they appear rather than allowing them to fester is liberating and energizing. Following the rules for self-care in fitness, diet, connectedness to people, and other features of well-being became the norm for our years in the desert.

We spent much time studying the teachings of religious leaders, both with each other and in groups. To imprint some of the intermediate lessons further into our living, we developed Spirit Pathways. The pathways consisted of seven major outdoors meditation sites equipped with chairs. Our visitors and we used these places, most in near-desert isolation, for meditation and communing with nature. The Spirit

Pathways reinforced the idea of committing to a vision and developing the will to carry this vision forward in our lives through right work, speech, and action.

Spirit Base Camp Impact

SBC was a place to expand on our spiritual nature, a place we honored not merely as our place to use but a place to build upon the beauty and serenity that already was present. We cleared out the broken and overgrown, groomed, tended, painted, and daily marveled at the beauty of the Sonoran Desert. We left about half of the place in its natural state, partly for its beauty but mostly for its function as a food source. Grazing quail and small critters, ever in danger of predators, need the food supplies and the cover of foliage for protection. We are, in many ways, part of that same food chain, and with that observation, we often wonder about the real meaning of life.

We chose to live an active life. We set out to enhance our learning with an emphasis on the creative. To do this, we focused on the observations and insights that come from spiritual practices of retreat, meditation, lingering in the twilight, using expressive arts of clay, painting, poetry, and walking. Our goal was to integrate ourselves into the fabric of the world around us. In these things, we felt closer to being in the presence of God. We saw SBC as a place of warmth and mystery that brought answers when we needed them, which guided us in our making, thinking, creating, and loving. SBC provided many transcendent moments for us.

We shared SBC widely, turning no one away. Many came—some often, others a few times—but none failed to receive the full hospitality of this magical place.

We set out to become neighbors in the best meaning of that term, and we succeeded. It was a deliberate action directed by instinct and professional knowledge and skills. It also was an act of love and a desire to connect as we had not done in other places. Before, our professional travel precluded close contact with neighbors. Here, we traveled little. We entrained ourselves to one another and SBC, and to neighbors we came to love and share with in our lives.

Spirituality to us evolved into these neighborly things and honoring the admonition to love your neighbor and do good and compassionate work. Doing this well required a renewed commitment to active aging. It meant living as though this time, right now, is Paradise.

We are called to live an active, purpose-filled life, and not just pray and imagine an afterlife filled with rewards. Life is the gift. We are called to live it fully NOW, AT THIS PRESENT TIME.

Our home now at Bishop Spencer Place is a village of people dedicated to Christian principles and serving others with kindness. The community forms around retirement years, but in many ways, it provides the kinds of connections and sharing noted in spiritual writings. In the early years of such communities, people lived much longer than anticipated. The spiritual nature of senior housing with a religious sponsor such as ours helps keep people going strong.

Portrait of Spiritually Active Aging People

What does all of this mean? After looking at our lives and studying some of the spiritual giants, sages, and wise people from many religious denominations and other cultures, here is a listing of the characteristics of an active spiritual ager:

- Their conduct is ethical, always telling the truth, showing up and focusing on positive outcomes. In their actions, they honor and respect others and pay attention to that which has heart and meaning.

- In their interactions with all creatures and events in the world, they do not harm, and they commit to helping others and embracing the world as it is.
- They focus daily on getting rid of obstacles to a full connection to the Spirit.
- They continually strive to be closer to God within them, being not-two with the God in All. In this dedication, they search for like-minded people on the same journey. Many find such companionship in organized religions.

Facing and Accepting Tough Realities

This discussion about religion and spirituality would not be complete without confronting the tough stuff we face now in our late eighties. We each have the privilege of living a blessed life with opportunities of experiencing a loving family, outstanding educational and professional opportunities, and marriage to a person who links with us in body, mind, and Spirit. We have been privileged to serve others through providing health care services, educating young professional students, organizing groups to make communities more productive, energizing people to get on with the good life, and challenging many to grow, develop, and become more spiritual.

Artificial knees and hips and a new heart valve, along with aches and pains, remind us that we have consumed too much food and not done enough exercise. We battle occasional memory lapses and give up driving because reflexes are slowing down. The litany is long.

However, in reality, we are fortunate that none of this is disabling. We worry about being the victim of cancer, diabetes, heart disease, stroke, or Alzheimer's. The assault on the elderly is unrelenting, and these problems are too prevalent not to get our attention. This reality changes our stance on life and gives us a feeling of fragility.

The most significant preoccupation we experience is with death. According to statistics, both of us are past our life expectancies. With each survived year, the expected used-by date is somewhat extended. However, we keep moving along with our lives. Our years of researching and engaging in active aging practices may well yield many more productive years. Therefore, periodic review of our effort is a practical use of time and energy. The spiritual aspects of life loom substantial near the end of our life.

Here in the continuing care community, we are surrounded by people who are experiencing all of the maladies we just cited. There are various departments of the nearby medical center to handle the progression of diseases prevalent in the elderly.

The health system is poised to respond to the needs of the elderly. Are we ready to do our part? Being more responsible for our health is not a new dimension and challenge for us. Much of what we need at this stage is within our power and will to supply, but it is up to us to focus and stay with our goals until the end. However, many look exclusively to the medical profession for answers and action.

There is one vital missing link between the elderly—all who use medical care, really—and the professionals. Our first contact with professionals presents that expert with an opportunity to assess our needs and to guide us on a path to wellness. But does the professional go beyond their requested or specialized service? Things like obesity are easily recognized by all professionals. Why not at this first contact say to the obese person; "It seems you have another issue that, if not addressed, often leads to severe medical problems such as diabetes and heart disease. The Medical Center offers a free introductory course on how to combat such issues; let me give you that information." Why not? Our health insurance system will pay for exams, but what we often need, and need early on, is proper education on health issues.

Why is this caveat about the medical system here in this text? We are called to call it out from our professional observation. It is a duty, one that could well be Spirit-inspired.

Our spiritual tasks from here out will be to continue to foster an abundant spiritual life and to acknowledge that the SPIRIT is calling us to give more entirely to others who are hurting from mental, psychological, and physical pain. We are being urged to contribute to the growth of the community we live in and spread the word about love, acceptance of life's burdens, and forgiveness of those who have wronged us. Now is the time for us to excel in becoming more fully functioning human beings, knowing that whatever happens is to be accepted.

We know that death is the harbinger of new life. Organized religion offers excellent specificity. In the end, organic growth stops, and inanimate matter is transformed and incorporated into the ongoing transformation of the planet in its relationship to the universe.

For Barbara, death is the beginning of an adventure for which she has prepared throughout her life. She needs to be in touch with the Spirit, grow in stillness and immediate compassion, and, finally, be open to all possibilities for becoming a completed work of the Spirit.

For Monty, death is a natural part of life. For him, the idea of "from dust to dust" is a reality. We come from, and belong to, the ongoing presence in the universe. It is as it is. Our job now is to do the best we can with what we have.

CHAPTER SIX (Q&A)

1.   But what if I don't believe there is a God out there who is looking out for me?

Good question. First, there is a lot of research that shows many positive health effects of religious practices. If you are intrigued by the idea of a Higher Being guiding the universe, talk to others who have a spiritual practice. Ask them about their beliefs about God. Ask if they pray regularly and whether this relationship with God gives them peace. If you continue to be interested in spiritual practice, visit and observe practices in a Christian church, Jewish synagogue, Buddhist temple, or other organized religious events.

Find out for yourself the benefits of cultivating an inward life with God, who loves you and cares for you. Having a long-term relationship with a life-giving Spirit buttresses you from the assaults of the everyday give-and-take. It also brings deep peace and courage for a person of faith, rooting them in the knowledge that God is present, watching over them and guiding their life. Having an inward experience and believing in connectedness to the more tremendous energies of the universe isn't restricted to belief in God. How this all relates is a mystery with theories abounding.

Many of the studies of long-lived populations show that fasting is common practice on religious holidays. Fasting also has positive health benefits. It is also a practical way to grow in self-discipline and mindfulness. Religions have rituals and gatherings as well as many social supports for their practitioners and adherents. Such social support has positive health benefits. Many of the standard practices within religions are practiced by others as well.

2. Are there other reasons to consider a religious or spiritual practice?

One reason stands out for us. Religions have moral codes that inculcate behaviors that are positive for society. One of the most famous is "Do unto others as you would have them do unto you." This is echoed in many religions and energizes people of faith to be sensitive to the needs of everyone around them. It tends to promote charity to others, offers refuge to the stranger, and provides food for the hungry and medicine to those ailing. Studies and admonitions point toward a positive health benefit for those who provide outreach and service to those in need. Some would argue that the giver may well benefit more than the recipient of charity. Would we have a caring society without such practices? Would these kinds of practices and values be promulgated and supported by other means? Perhaps. We don't know, but we give great credit to religion and spirituality for what they promote and for their contribution to a good society.

Indeed, we might argue for another benefit as well. In considering what is appropriate behavior toward the one in need, it is imperative to ask oneself: *If I were in the same circumstance, is this something that would be of benefit to me, or would it possibly be hurtful?* Close introspection might lead to this question: Is it better to give the person a fish for food or to teach them how to fish? Would I be better off relying on gifts and charity of others or working harder to fend for myself?

Introspection of this nature might lead to a nuanced answer rather than a dualistic either/or response. For instance, perhaps it is best to feed a person first and teach them self-reliance later. Or, in some cases, long-term support for a person who is learning and strengthening needs to occur to help them move from poverty to independence. Families may need years of help to get out of debt.

And it may be necessary to educate both children and parents at the same time.

3. **What other ways might one gain some of the benefits of religions and spirituality discussed here?**

Meditation is often mentioned as a practice to still the mind to relieve stress. Religious people and mystics use meditation to achieve a sense of transcendence.

4. **Are religion and spirituality the only two ways to live an ethical life in community with others?**

Hardly. Monty doesn't remember during childhood ever having anyone discuss spirituality with him. Nor was it a subject in Barbara's more religious family. Over the years, we have had grown more spiritual. This reflects more a meeting of the minds on the meaning of spiritual with less reference to or commitment to rules and edicts of a formal church connection. It comes from being exposed to more thinking about living a good life dedicated to service much in the tradition of religious-sponsored organizations. Although many hospitals we worked with were sponsored by religious organizations, some were purely secular yet with the same dedication to serving the sick and poor. Many groups and organizations have no explicit connect to religion or spirituality but do much of the same kind of work with similar motivations and dedication.

Connection to the universal notions of love and service comes in many flavors and guises. Underneath it all is the same family—the human family, the family of Life and Love.

CHAPTER SEVEN

Social Factors: Stronger Together

Social creatures we are

Responsible for ourselves

Born into families

Bonded in nature

Rooted in friendships and community

Love and Compassion are nature's healers

Be present to others

Love yourself

Reach out and serve

Health benefits galore

Caring attracts caring

Build networks

Serve other

Serve yourself

Love the family,

Treat your neighbor as yourself

Introduction

Being close to others, having a life partner, is one way of becoming more fully oneself. Human beings are more than single energy fields; we thrive on proximity to others. Aloneness rarely works well for long. Yes, a solo adventure into the wilderness is often shown to be a coming-of-age ritual. It helps the individual to realize their own strengths. It cements the truth that our bodies, minds, and spirits are intact. And, a solo venture can work to provide a life always pushing into the future. But life isn't fully complete without companionship. Even the method for procreation requires two sets of DNA, not one. Why? One from a single line isn't as strong as a combination of two cell lines. Many lives are strengthened when two are joined in friendship, fellowship, or marriage. Many bonding opportunities exist, many lives are enriched in this manner. So our comments on social issues come from a strong sense of bonding with another, and, its importance based upon our experiences, observations and reading of the literature on health and wellness.

Importance of Human Contact

The frequent loss of family members and acquaintances is a significant challenge of aging. Continuing to build relationships during this process is vital to a healthy active aging process.

Positive relations and frequent interaction with other people are plus factors in promoting good health. Good ties with family and colleagues at work as well as play and learning are invaluable. Shared affection is one of the most positive experiences one can have. In our spiritual traditions, the ideal is to worship together, sing together, eat together, love one another, bond, and go through life together. *Together* has many meanings, and there are ways to enhance the bonding among people.

Relationships are often the key ingredient to achieving agreement among competing interests by finding ways to cooperate for win-win outcomes. Having a good trainer for fitness, a companion to share the journey of walking or dieting, or someone to share a tennis or bridge game—these are essential elements in success. Good social relations permeate the lives of those whose aging travels a smoother road.

For those whose aging is burdened by disease, good relations can mean the difference between despair and a good day. Having a visitor on a bad day can make life better. Animals also can be a great pick-me-up for those impaired by illness or just the ravages of age. Of course, such contacts also are positive for the fit and vital.

> **The best way to describe the importance of social contacts is to watch a baby react with wonder and positive emotion, to feel the caress of a human or the nudging from a friendly puppy.**

Humans share one of our most essential characteristics—our genes—with another. Why might that be? The most appealing theory is that our own gene pool, over a life span, accumulates many errors. Two or more gene pools make for more ideas and more options, more advantages, and more defenses against failure and loss.

The second critical relationship is with the host—the mother—nurturing that new life and all the biomes that come with her body. If the fetus survives to birth, a human begins a journey, growing until adulthood and then slowly declining to old age.

After our emergence from our mother's womb, life gets more complicated. Others come to see us in our infancy. Some sing and cuddle, and the young life gets a lift and hug, soothing words, and welcoming formation experience. A presence of bonding, good social relations, and strong family ties contributes to a life of growth. Early failures to get the needed feedback from many others besides the mother negatively impacts the young life.

Social Relationships

Positive experiences of interacting with others can be a plus for good health. This should start early in life. Such experiences can lead to such things as a better job or learning a critical skill that sets a career on track. Early adverse experiences can cause a train wreck.

There will be many ups and downs through the course of life. Imagine the results if a young child is put in front of a TV to watch shows instead of having an adult or older sibling take them out to run and play in a park. Consider the differences that might evolve for some-one given piano lessons, monitored and guided in well-defined practice, in contrast to getting lessons and left on your own to practice or not.

Childhood can't be relived. What we have is what was available— genetics, childrearing, schooling—and that is what we must live with and optimize. Life isn't all roses and nectar for most of us. But what we have can be improved and shaped. Once that is accepted and learned, the world has much to offer. In health, there is much that can be pre-vented or reversed if one is willing to learn. We have seen it happen and done it ourselves.

People of all ages can grow and learn. Growing and gaining exper-tise requires sound starts on how to do things, insights into what to practice and how to practice, and feedback on how one is performing. Many things we attribute to ideal childrearing and learning experience come from our relations with parents, teachers, and coaches. This is as true for adults as for children.

Active aging is best done by those who cultivate healthy relationships.

Not every relationship is healthy. We often are advised to avoid relationships that drag us down. This dragging can be the tension cre-ated by negative people. It can come from anyone, including individuals who might well be perfectly compatible with others. The factors that matter are those that are important to each individual.

If we seek advice, counsel, and/or training to learn and grow, we need someone with expert knowledge and skills in the field we wish to study. That assistance doesn't need to be the best in an area, but it does need to be of more exceptional skill and knowledge than we possess. And over time, it may require us to seek other teachers as our own level of performance improves. If we seek growth in a skill, it is probable that we will have many different coaches as we progress. Ready to train for a new level? Obtain qualified resources to assist you.

We tend to prefer companions with similar interests. Even within families where the bonds stretch over decades and stem from many similar life experiences, friction can develop. In families, we naturally feel an obligation to get along. When parents are gone, those bonds tend to be rationalized more as "she or he is my only family left." Over time, many of the rough edges smooth out, and affection remains. Having those ties can promote health and well-being.

Social Relations and Health

Adults who are more socially connected are healthier and live longer than their more-isolated peers.

Social isolation can result in psychological and physical dis-integration and even death. Jails use separation as a form of punishment. Other key findings of the impact of social relations on health include impacts:

- on behavioral, psychosocial, and physiological pathways
- costs and benefits
- relationships which shape health outcomes

- cost and benefits not distributed evenly in the population.

Partner with Someone Who Brings Out Your Best Behaviors

Choosing partners and friends whose behaviors are positive will help you in improving your own habits. Perhaps the reverse might happen—choosing a partner whose habits you can change. On the other hand, a partner who drops a bad habit such as smoking is likely to influence his or her partner to do the same.

Once upon a time, as such stories go, Monty was a cigar smoker. His office, home, and work . . . well, reeked of it. Once, in a meeting he was asked to leave to smoke. After a few such hints, and, really for him, the ease of quitting took over. Without the friendly persuasion and suggestions of others, however, who knows? He might still be smoking the stogies and pipes. Leaving a habit behind isn't easy, and support for the change is always helpful.

It is difficult to help others when we don't really know ourselves very well. So before jumping to help, be sure you have the right answers to these kinds of questions.

- What is it about you that might be good for a friend, for a partner, or for a teacher and coach?
- What about us will be right for the other? Should we find ways to overcome our shortcomings or shy away from people whose lives may not be better if we seek closeness?

Our answers to these kinds of questions are few, if any, but the items need to be considered in seeking out, establishing, and benefiting from social contacts and relationships.

As we begin to think seriously about active aging for ourselves, our lives already have been shaped by a variety of social connections going back to conception, birth, childhood, schooling, marriage, careers, and more. With longer lives, it may be best to consider working on a new life plan rather than merely tweaking existing habits. Our appreciation for the need for good social relations was in all of our retirement plans, but upon retirement in Tucson, we ramped up our involvements to do more to organize our neighborhood to facilitate better social connectedness.

Social relations are essential throughout life, and social isolation is more likely after leaving the world of paid employment. Those we know from professional connections, suppliers, and customers, often are among our closest friends. When leaving the workplace, one departs from the regular routines with many friends and finds themselves the next day at home, just among family, or, perhaps worse, if no family or friends, just alone.

Our Experience

Our situation was different since our last paid for work years were conducted from home. We had home offices and saw clients at their workplaces and professional colleagues mostly at national meetings. Our back-office work was contracted out, so our downsizing preceded our retirement. One day we closed our business, movers took some office things and records, and our apartment was emptied. We drove to Arizona, leaving behind an icy rain as we said goodbye to our Washington, DC, home and our professional careers. Sunshine aplenty awaited in Arizona. It was a new world. We knew no one in our chosen new home—no close friends, no close professional colleagues, and no coaches to help us begin this new life.

A local church offered social connections, and, with time, our personal relations multiplied. Networks always exist, so as we stayed open to new people new relationships formed. As is often the case, some of the members at the church we attended were also our neighbors, and those connections led to others.

Our commitment to fitness also led to other social connections, including walkers and the occasional horseback riders who lived nearby. We met a lot of new people while walking our dogs. Dog lovers are always to be found and easy to meet and greet.

We had planned to continue some professional work when we moved to Arizona. For Monty, it led to a part-time teaching assignment. For Barbara, it was a nurse refresher course and a part-time job for a hospice organization. Barbara met more people in her course and Monty dipped back into graduate education for health administration.

Before long, we decided that neither of our employment options was satisfactory. What caused these long considered goals to be unsatisfactory? Barbara enjoyed the work with patients but soon the management asked her to do more project work using her in-depth consulting skills, something she wanted to leave behind. For Monty it was partly a locational problem, i.e., the class was 100 miles from home and posed commuting problems. Another factor might have been the fact that we didn't take a sufficient break from quitting our consulting practice and going back into work. Or perhaps we underestimated the dropping back to more mundane work was itself a problem? Perhaps we weren't expecting the drop in status and the too easy nature of the work. Whatever were the reasons, not staying in professional health care occupations opened major opportunities for us to pursue social and creative interest long neglected.

We settled in our neighborhood. Barbara began to work on social connectivity and organization in addition to art and spiritual practices. Monty began by joining and creating hiking groups to build on one of his dreams. Both did clay work which for Monty morphed into acrylic painting which became a major outlet for his creative energies. However, 9/11,2001 came, the use of airplanes to bomb the Twin Tower in New York City and the Pentagon in Washington, DC. Within weeks we re-engaged in health care as volunteers in emergency response with federal, state and local agencies as well as in our neighborhood. After a few weeks, we were recruited to help establish a Medical Reserve Corps, participate in a Citizen's Corps Council, and more. While the terror attacks on 9/11/2001 were the stimulus for these new organizations, the efforts took an all-disasters approach, so we trained for many new roles and met great people in the process.

Planning Ahead

We had friends in other parts of Arizona and looked there for possible places to live. However, our main criteria were fitness, outdoor hiking, and proximity to proper medical care. And even those friends we sought out were not involved in the kinds of activities we sought to revitalize our lives, to be more active. The life style we sought was different from that of our retired friends who played golf and tennis, hit the cocktail circuit and long dinner parties.

We settled on an area where we could actually walk from our house into Saguaro National Park, a federally designated wilderness area with human use limited to designated trails. By picking the place to live, we also were choosing to live among people who shared our interest in being outdoors, in nature, and in hiking. No doubt those wanting to live in a golf-oriented community seek both golf and like-minded people.

We picked the ideal area for our fitness and lifestyle purposes. It was a square-mile area that initially expected to become part of the Saguaro National Park. Some of the first people we met were walking with their dogs in the neighborhood. They soon became our guides to the mountain trails.

There were no neighborhood organizations for us to join. Instead, we set out to begin our walks in the neighborhood. Our fitness adventure began, and our effort to connect with others soon blossomed. We first met the horses, dogs, javelina (similar to wild boars), and occasional rattle snakes along the roadways. Then, one or two at a time, we met people and got to know them as we shared stories and eventually became closer. Over time, we visited each other's homes.

Advancements in our social networking came when one neighbor asked if we would help form a neighborhood watch. Ours was not a high-crime area, but the park attracted a lot of traffic and the occasional robber. We agreed to help, and Barbara first led the steering committee, then later the Neighborhood Watch—a Sheriff's Department-sponsored organization. After we joined many meetings with neighbors, our acquaintances became friends and good neighbors. One project led to another.

At one point, someone in the neighborhood wanted to convert a home to a treatment center. The house could have been ideal for that but the project would have significantly changed the character of the neighborhood. Like most such neighborhoods with unique features to protect, we helped organize the fight to block that development. To engage such events, we hosted a neighborhood association. Engaging, working, and sharing our organizational expertise, we built strong ties with neighbors. Helping and being concerned for others are significant ways to become and stay socially connected.

Investing Time and Energy

Community service also connected us and our professional skills to others whose needs we could help meet and who shared their love, knowledge, and talents with us. Our faith in social bonding through the community was well rewarded. Helping out is our way of investing in the community.

After the 9/11/2001 terror attacks came the ramping up of homeland security. Shortly after, a neighbor for whom we had helped build the Notch Neighborhood Watch organization asked if we would help create a Medical Reserve Corps. We agreed, and Barbara managed the recruitment and training task for clinicians to help with immunizations.

Monty joined AmeriCorps full time to help create and staff the Medical Reserve Corps.

Serving others is a great way to meet one's need for social connection and to benefit from stronger social ties. Serving is its own reward. Our service to the community was often noted, although experiencing the connections and honoring our life purpose of helping people was more than sufficient. While building social connectivity, volunteering strengthens one mentally, physically, psychologically, and spiritually. It also makes you a more desirable neighbor, friend, and citizen.

Changing Retirement Locations

We left our desert retreat in Tucson to live at Bishop Spencer Place in the center of Kansas City. Our plan for moving to such a place was in part to be prepared when or if a medical crisis hit. As we prepared to move, with air tickets purchased to come to Kansas City to buy into a CCRC, an unexpected heart artery bypass and valve replacement for Monty was ordered. That event made the switch more difficult but didn't change our new direction.

Leaving our desert retreat home meant leaving associations we had helped organize. Many people we met remain good friends. We also moved from the great outdoors, where communing with nature was a primary daily activity. In the city, everything is organized, and services are purchased and supplied by workers. Here one learns how to live mostly indoors and to navigate among the many services and richly endowed cultural features of a great city. Each environment presents challenges. We believe that by making a major change in our living environment, we give ourselves the kind of problems that will keep us actively engaging in new social connections.

Moving from the desert to the city means finding new friends, a relatively easy thing to do here where we live close to many others. Here, we all share similar concerns, such as the desire to be in a tightly knit community—a community that is prepared to help with our growing needs for more services. It turns out that the most essential function in this community isn't one offered for money but the companionship and friendship of close neighbors. In Tucson, we had to build a lot of the structures needed to have an actual neighborhood. Here, many neighborhood structures already exist. Everyone is welcomed and in a short time becomes a member of a close family of friends.

One problem many seniors face is memory loss, and for some the ultimate loss is to Alzheimer's disease. Like for so many diseases, one recommendation is to stay active and around people. In retirement communities, one is aware that many suffer some memory loss. Our fitness classes have a variety of people, and those with memory losses often are star performers. They function well doing exercises

Exercise helps strengthen our brains, and doing it with others satisfies our human need for social interactions.

Those who are married or living in a committed relationship have an advantage—companionship. Others keep their favorite pets, which nurture them as the pets are nurtured by the resident. Fellowship is vital. Many singles find others who will provide mutual support and assistance. In these congregate living communities, people become acquainted and develop ties quickly.

Finding and Keeping Friends

Some people join a retirement community and then find every excuse not to participate in the many activities planned for residents. We did our early exercise work at a nearby hospital as part of a cardiac fitness program. It wasn't long before we realized that this group of clinicians and patients were becoming friends. We enjoyed their company, we admired their work, and we applauded our fellow exercisers on their progress. When the formal program was finished, we elected to stay on and work out with this same group. Eventually, we left to meet our needs beyond what was offered, but we keep in touch and will use these clinicians for periodic evaluations. We have friends there now. One of our fellow Bishop Spencer Place (BSP) residents actually moved here to continue his own exercise at the cardiac exercise location we used. There he had friendships and support for his efforts.

We moved from that rehabilitation exercise program to join various classes offered here at BSP. Over time, we've found ourselves spending more time with fellow classmates, having dinners with them, and chatting when we meet in the halls or at events. It isn't hard to find friends if you open up to the opportunities offered for group activities. The exercise programs themselves provide the essential opportunities to grow, but in time comes a need to find further challenges. All group functions offer opportunities to increase and improve upon your social connections.

The life-enrichment program here offers periodic trips to events, exceptional restaurants, and parks. We have met and become close friends with people initially encountered on these trips. We also are exploring features of this sophisticated city culture that provide ideas for further growth and, no doubt, still other new social connections.

Finding people you might like to have as friends is a significant first step, but building a relationship requires more. Remember birthdays, which is easy to do here, because a list of them is published every month. Dinners and cocktail get-togethers are easy to do when dining out is a daily affair. Similarly, seek new acquaintances to attend an event, and make it a point to connect. Time and connections will build bridges, and, for many, that will cement relationships.

Relationship-Forming Risks

Social relationships can be toxic as well as life-enhancing, so it helps to have a choice. A young man Monty met at college and just out of a prep school in New England said, "I don't try to make friends early. It takes a while to sort out who I might really want as a friend." Sound advice. Both of us had careers where our jobs and school assignments, not a personal choice, defined our social circles, and many friendships came from those encounters as well. That helped form a broader picture of humanity than our own decisions might have.

However, taking care to avoid quick personal impressions also is a wise thing to do. We urge caution in this because someone who isn't impressive at first eventually may deepen our own experience of humanity's vast range of peoples and cultures. After a while, the old saying "I have never met a stranger" seems apt. Openness to knowing others is a powerful stimulant to help us become a better person through encounters across a wider swath of humanity.

> **Use the advice to young carpenters: "measure twice, cut once"; it pays to be thoughtful about choosing friends.**

Measure often, chose wisely; this holds true in many social situations. For instance, it helps to take time to visit more than one church to see how each measures up to your expectations. This clearly applies to marriage as well. For our generation, marriage is a once-in-a-lifetime choice. For Monty, that didn't work out well the first time around. However, the second time, with a bit more wisdom, things worked very well indeed.

In selecting neighbors, our first choice is rarely based on the people but more on location and whether other criteria are met. Later comes another sorting out—who is open to new relationships, and which of those seem most compatible?

Neighbors eventually sort out along affinity lines, but care needs to be taken not to give offense or, if done, to mend the fence soon. Neighbors, like family, are there for a long time. The same care should be taken to sort out potential friendships in the retirement communities. It soon will become apparent who is interested most in things that interest you. Contacts will happen, and things may flow smoothly from there.

Relationships can become toxic because not everyone may welcome the same kind of friendship. Some desire close and relatively exclusive relations. Others have a wide range of friends with whom they may desire connections for different reasons. Sports, movies, music, fitness, and politics are examples of patterns people follow. Be easy to know, but do not allow toxic relations to continue. Some connections can't be severed but need not become exclusive or even frequent. A retirement community is a small neighborhood where almost everyone encounters each other many times a week.

Improving Social Connections

Planned and unplanned opportunities exist to change one's life circumstances to enhance careers and retirement. Consider breaking up how work-life proceeds. Perhaps continue substantially longer in jobs to earn money for later retirement and stay engaged in a career. Obviously, this will keep friends and colleagues close. This also will become more necessary as people live longer and healthier lives. The idea of working longer already is a reality for many and will be for a majority by the end of this century.[16] At age 50, Monty went to law school to enhance

---

16   The Bureau of Labor Statistics provides the best data on workers ages and trends. When Social Security ages for retirement at 62 and 65, those years were about the same as upper limits of life. Now with workers retiring at 62, they may well live until 79, with 17 years of retirement. Some will make it twice that

his work knowledge and found new friends and connections. Barbara, near age 50, earned a degree in Transpersonal Psychology, learned new methods, enhanced her consulting practice, and made friends outside our regular health care work. Age 50 is a young age to begin a new career. In law school, a classmate of Monty's was past 60 and planning a joint practice with a daughter of his who was in our class as well. At age 65 he could easily practice law for another 30 years.

If working longer at the same job isn't attractive, consider another career that might well begin before the current retirement age occurs. Another option is to volunteer. One neighbor who had run a business found satisfaction transporting patients at a Veteran's Administration hospital. Another friend found work-shelving products in a store to stay active and fit. Being an orderly at a hospital or stock clerk can avoid much of the inaction that often occurs for retirees. We found productive volunteer work building structures and programs for Homeland Security. Our neighborhood development jobs were similar.

Our retirement move to Bishop Spencer Place is going in the same direction. Our first priority is keeping fit so we can enjoy our mobility and intellectual stimulation, and doing so means engaging in the life of the community. Our volunteer work is growing as we settle into our new digs and lifestyle. Fortunately, social connections grow fast here.

Important Things to Remember

One thing that stands out for us is the need to have a role in the life around us. Service is at the core of the health professions. Using our skills in some fashion remains essential. Helping and being engaged in serving remains at the center of our lives. Having a purpose in life makes things worth doing, and volunteering offers this. Continuing to

---

number and for many their life savings gone before they are even near to that age. Income will drive some back into the labor force, and for many, boredom will lead them to work. Those post retirement jobs are often self employment or part time.

work at a profession or any activity that keeps us engaged is helpful. This is what it means to have a strong sense of purpose. Having an overarching goal in life gives meaning. It also provides a solid reason for the harder work of fitness, keeping skills up to date, and going the extra mile in helping others. We consider it a duty to help others and to invest forward to make life better for all, something often called Paying Back for our own blessings. It is a gift to be able to help others, something for which we are grateful.

The social networks for many will be around their places of worship. For others, it may be a social group to which they have belonged for years. And for others, a charity provides social interaction. Some find it in military and work connections. Whatever the connection, it pays to stay active, be in touch, and help if and when you can.

One of the oldest things to remember is the Golden Rule: Do unto others as you would have them do unto you, or the reverse: Do not do to others that which you don't want them to do to you.

Doing good is life-enhancing for both the giver and the recipient. The giver often is rewarded with a more positive self-image when doing good for others.

Social networks can be robust. People in their nineties who share a meal or a drink in the pub with friends from kindergarten enjoy a social connection of great value. Studies of long-lived peoples often comment on the social networks that are fed frequently, sometimes daily, for a lifetime. Having one or more groups that meet regularly and share the burdens and joys of life is a strong asset for those who seek to live actively.

Ample opportunities are available to reach out a bit and make new friends, volunteer, help someone in need, or find a new interest to pursue. More-extroverted persons can do these things naturally, while introverts find it more difficult. If friendship comes slowly, the old standby idea really does work: fake it until you make it work. Don't give up quickly, and if it takes a lot more tries, evaluate what you are doing, improve on the approach, and try, try again.

Although we haven't found many scientific studies that mention this, we've found that bringing some fun and joy to every encounter is useful and rewarding. If you want to enjoy life, try to offer others a bit of laughter, a good mood, and a friendly face to lift their spirits. Yours will be lifted as well, and others will welcome encounters with you.

Isolation can be debilitating and even deadly. Avoid becoming a recluse. Getting out and being with others is necessary and makes for a much more balanced day. When others benefit from entering into social relations because you reached out, life is even better.

On the other hand, a degree of isolation and quiet reflective time can be useful for anyone, just as a good party, some music or a film or a dinner party is good for us all. The key is to have all in good measure, in good time, and with good friends and family. Stay connected to other people.

CHAPTER SEVEN (Q&A)

1. **Those who move around a lot over a career realize the process of being alone and finding new friends is endless. Is this a challenge for you? What are some of the ways to deal with it?**

Living includes some moments in time when we glide by ourselves and other moments when we stand side by side with others. The presence of others at home, in our work life, and during rest and relaxation adds to the joy of being human. Sharing stories, secrets, and life goals with others reinforces our resolve to live life to its fullest.

No doubt moving around and experiencing disruptions in social connections presents hurdles for long-term relationships. New careers in professions like ours (mostly health administration) often means that the people one sees and works with are from different parts of the country. Academics often work in collaboration with others from multiple states. Many professionals, over time, work in different places as they progress in the profession. When retiring, they may or may not be near people with whom they have worked. So yes, it is a challenge of if one can make new friends easily, a easy problem to solves, make new friends.

In retirement, the people in one's orbit are likely to be neighbors living nearby, and, for those in retirement places, those who dine together tend to run in the same circles. Hobbies may also be shared along with social events. Friendship and interaction patterns can flourish. However, unlike persons who live in the same town throughout life, friendships and confidences are likely more short-term in retirement communities. In our community, for example, most of the people are relatively new to us. But for some neighbors in their nineties, their friends here today may have been in kindergarten with them! With proximity, there is the potential of forming close friendships stemming from interest in some shared activity such as bridge, exercise, opera, or jazz.

When lifelong friends aren't present, get out and do enjoyable things. Find those who share your interest, and go from there. If relations aren't positive, move on. Find others to share the fun and downsides in your life and in their lives as well.

2. Living in the desert with significant distance between neighbors made casual opportunities for visiting difficult. How does that differ from living now in a retirement community apartment?

It's night-and-day different. In the desert, many days might pass without seeing a neighbor. Even days when we hiked the neighborhood or went on into the nearby park, we didn't necessarily encounter a neighbor. In contrast, in apartment living with many others of similar age and with a range of abilities, we see dozens of people daily at different events. We can much more easily socialize in the apartment living: We share exercise classes with some. In our casual take-out and sit-down food service area, we encounter many of the same people daily in addition to the friendly staff. In more formal dining, we have the opportunity to visit with others. It is actually challenging to be a loner in such facilities. And when anyone who does tend to stay isolated, others are likely to offer to join them for visiting, dining, exercising, or going to some other communal event. Anyone wanting to increase their social activities will find ample opportunities where seniors live close together.

Social connections seem generally desirable. Are there more critical times when connectivity is vital? Yes, any time one is vulnerable, having someone to share the burden of doubt, fear, or concern can be stress reducing.

3. **Social support is very important, but when illness strikes, there is no substitute for full-time, trained help. If this is true, why all the emphasis on social connections?**

    Health care professionals and all types of caregivers are needed from time to time. But the voice of a companion, a close friend, or even a friendly visitor seeking to provide comfort is a valuable addition to the fabric of life. And the value of being the friend and not the one in need of solace is ample and equally valid. Giving comfort, being a friendly visitor, adds benefits to life: social inter-action, life affirmations, love, and kindness are life-enhancing for all parties. So yes, professional full-time help is essential but not a substitute for the friendship and interactions with others.

4. **Is everyone always open to having friends or being friendly? This all seems a little preachy to me.**

    No, you are right; some people do not mix well with others. We don't find everyone open to positive ongoing relations with us. This doesn't happen often, but it does happen. And some people who might want to be friendly are not always someone with whom we might want to spend more time. That happens too. We don't see this as more or less than the human condition. We cannot expect a good match for friendship with everyone. There are times when we do the rejecting or avoidance and times when it is another way. Life happens.

5. **Social support as presented here seems to focus mostly on how it benefits me. Isn't it something of a two-way street?**

    Much of the literature on health issues seem to focus on why one benefits from having social support. And in our society we focus a lot on having governmental programs for support of people who need help. Most of the nation's hospitals and social agencies were privately organized, often by religious groups, to support neighbors in need. Religions stress helping the neighbor. Helping others is also seen in religions to be the good works that help the helper in their own relations with God. And there is good evidence that doing good things for others is good for the giver as well.

But it isn't exactly a two-way street. If A provides help for B, the good that comes to A may well be from other sources, including sources anticipated by religions as well as psychological feelings occurring but not attributed to the benefit occurring for B nor any action on B's part. Sounds a bit complicated, doesn't it? Because it is. The actions of A and B are often one-way in transactional human terms, but the impacts on both A and B, while seemingly separate in direct causation, occur in tandem, one after another.

Those whose religions stress service believe that the rewards are from God; those who may be more spiritually inclined but who do not attribute all to God may well see such apparent reciprocity as being the way the universe works. "What goes around comes around" is one saying along this line.

6. Are there other aspects of social support you have studied but do not discuss here?

Yes, there are several. In our consulting practice, we often found that many ideas for moving forward came out in group and interview situations. We believe that multiple brains and minds working in concert with similar issues stimulate thoughts that might not otherwise be formulated or considered by either of the parties.

In other fields of study, we have noted that electrical and magnetic fields exist and, no doubt, intersect in social situations. These fields may well trigger thoughts that might not otherwise be thought or, if considered, might be different. Thus, in our consulting work, we always considered the end product to be the work of many, not merely those who write it all up for presentation.

CHAPTER EIGHT

Your Active Aging Toolkit

Where do you want to go?
How will you steer your life?
Many choices to be made
Problem-solving tools exist
Find the right ones
Steer a faithful course

If one day something shows up
And the message is CHANGE COURSE
Fear not, life offers many pathways
A few right ones are there for you

Need refreshing? Fix a good meal
Take a vacation, go back to school
Build your own business
Life is an adventure
Keep learning
Invest in yourself, grow and flourish
Live in the present, focus attention
Act on what can be done . . . Today!!

Build and Use Your Tool Kit

Sometimes we are self-directed researchers, and, at other times, we are learners and teachers. In much of our work, we wrestle with ideas instead of building and fixing tangible objects or serving individual patients. However, we understand how important it is to use the right tool for the job. Although most of us have tried it, hammering in a screw is never as effective as using a screwdriver.

We share the toolkit we used in writing this book because the tools worked for us and may be helpful for others. You may not need every tool right now, but they will be waiting when you do. These are our most-used tools.

Face it. None of us gets to pick the gene pool from which to begin life, so the issue is how to live the life we have. Ample tools and methods are available for sorting out the kinds of choices we must make to enhance our life and make it the active life that we desire. If the lottery of life didn't cause enough variation, our growing up in different cultures and with such a variety of circumstances makes things even more varied. Variety isn't bad or wrong, but it makes the teaching and advice business difficult. We are—in so many ways, each and every one of us—unique. Yes, we share much but not everything. So we must each adapt what we have to what life offers.

**Success requires dealing with our
unique selves.**

Ideally, each of us should develop healthy habits early and practice them for life, which makes our experience an active one. Play and curiosity then are combined with fun, and all is nurtured by loving parents, neighbors, friends, teachers, and others who play roles in our lives as well. Whatever path we take, at some point it occurs to most of us that someday we will need to be prepared for retirement. Recognizing that such ideal happenings are more dreams than reality, we need to design our lives to meet our ideas for an active life.

The big issue that first attracted our attention was the need to think about how to finance retirement. Our experience in finance was mostly our prudent habits of spending what we could afford based on our current income. Earning in the early years of life would be necessary for many reasons, such as for treats or even necessities, but ultimately for making independent choices. Only with the teen years did questions of saving for college or other longer-term investment decisions arise. We believe strongly that higher education is a substantial investment in human capital—namely, yourself and your abilities. This ideal didn't jell for Monty until he served in the military but earlier for Barbara, whose parents were college educated.

We married in our early forties, and neither had any saved capital. Our academic careers were beginning. We had management education and knew about the magic of compound interest on saving, but savings were missing. We had human capital in abundance, and that needed to be used to acquire retirement resources. Moreover, we worked for universities that provided pension plans that vest from day one, not after many years of service. Those few years in academic work provided a base for retirement.

Live in the Present

So as we began our married life, both over forty, we had no savings but lots of human capital. We were trained and had good job prospects. Aside from neither of us being expert in the field of finance, we had skills in planning, evaluating, and decision tools, which are as useful for individuals as for organizations. So we had to find ways to go forward with nearly half of our working and earning years already behind us and no savings for the future.

Where does one begin such a journey? Begin with where you are right now, in the present. We were both just out of our most recent educational adventure and were ready to pursue academic careers. We could not change our past, but we could find things to do in the present if we chose focus there. Working on long-range planning and later evaluating the plan doesn't work well. So, what we could we do today about the many tomorrows that may come? Plan, save, stay fit, and keep learning. Every goal inherently has within it small steps that we can do today.

We are in the present, and this is the best place to design or plan for an active life. Indeed, we actually can take concrete action in the present that provides the first test of our ideas about how to proceed.

This idea of living fully in the present is powerful. Right now, you can have an idea and begin working on it. For example, once on a Friday, we were in a class where we were asked to share a goal that we would do something about in the next week. Monty said he would begin working out two days a week at a nearby gym. He said he was confident at a ten level (the highest confidence) that it would happen. However, it was too time-consuming after a few months, so he re-designed his exercise schedule to better use in-house resources. Begin with trial and error, and evaluate whether it's working or not. If not, move on to the next best option. Now Monty works out six days a week, with four of those being two hours or more in length. Life and opportunities will change leading to a change in goals, but the time to begin a new journey or shift is right now, in the present.

When Monty returned home from class, that Friday he arranged for transportation the following week and selected Tuesday and Thursday for his gym workouts. Further, he arranged to get an assessment to begin the new journey on Thursday. It was easy. Yes, it had been a possibility for several years. Yes, it was often a stated goal. However, it was a goal in the air, not concrete, not a hard decision. Hard decisions are possible today, but they rarely work when made as something to be done in the nebulous future. Now, we are more likely to have an idea, discuss it, and then before ending the discussion, ask what can we do to begin this now. Research and planning to give it more in-depth consideration aren't ruled out, but we pursue it in the present before the impetus for change dissipates.

An action orientation in life is important. Time taken bemoaning actions not taken earlier really are a waste of effort.

How many times have you heard someone say, "I wish I had done that earlier. Am I too old for that"? The problem often is not the time left to reap huge benefits from taking the considered action; it is that many have a fixed idea about what it takes for success in life.

Too many people assume that life is controlled entirely by their genes. For others, the factors controlling one's life is the lack of money, position, or education of their parents. In truth, one can begin a new phase in life right now, this very day. The past is gone. In economic terms, the past financial decisions should not dictate present choices. Whatever happened before is gone. What is before us in the present moment is an opportunity. How we deal with opportunity determines whether it is productive or wasted. No decision is a huge decision, because procrastination will waste the day, our bodies will age, and that moment in time will have come and gone.

Keep Your Sense of Play

Remember how open you were as a child, with lots of curiosity and wonderment with time for play and exploration? Keep building your resources for being as creative as a playful child. There are dozens of ways to proceed with making this point. Because life is that which is happening right now, in the present, it makes sense to believe and act as if the ideas and tools we need are at hand for creative living, right now, right here, in the present.

Be Guided by Goals

We credit design ideas for keeping our thinking grounded. We act on what is in front of us. We used this approach often in our work. We have used it for our personal lives as well. The method seeks to help people mentally model possible pathways by ideation and building prototype options for testing. Mentally modeling ideas is a wonderfully productive method for creating new realities for oneself.

Monty got interested in law by being involved with mergers and other aggregations of hospitals. He met lawyers, served as an expert witness, and found lawyers at every stage of significant institutional change. So he decided to learn their craft to do his current work more comprehensively. It worked well since to change institutional behavior often requires legal and policy changes embedded in law and customs that mimic civil laws. This fairly intense use of ideation, mental modeling, and noodling about the prospects for using tools or knowing different things and how they might be useful prepares the mind for taking steps, sometimes substantial one, in new directions. To an observer, it might seem precipitous to take such measures. Radical as they might seem, the measures are often well thought out in concept making the marshaling of energy needed to accomplish them more easily obtained.

In addition to mentally modeling, seeking out people in the roles we aspire to play works well also. We have met many successful hospital executives over the years who got their start by first interviewing people who were holding jobs of possible interest. Many landed entry jobs for experience before entering into graduate programs to prepare for top positions. Many of those connections paid off for years, with move after move associated with advice from an early interviewee who became a trusted mentor. It's a method that works. It's called building out your life. We are where we are. There are ways to go, some ideation and analysis help to know where to look, and people to see. Instead of just writing things down, engage areas of interest.

Maintain a Bias for Action

Time is precious. Don't put off until tomorrow what you can do today. Time lost to procrastination, daydreaming, or avoiding decisions is a real cost. Time is something we cannot bank and save for another day. We use it in the present or lose it. How many times do you say, "Let me make a note of that" and then forget it? Alternatively, day after day, you think of things you might do and occasionally talk about them but never act on them.

The scope of our ideas can be an obstacle to action, such as if one seeks to travel the world in a few weeks or months. Getting around will take lots of time. Experiencing even a few places is difficult without weeks on the ground. Want to travel? Planning is required, and it can begin with a list of things to do, many of which can be done the day the idea emerges. Collecting information on ways to accomplish your travel goals; getting on mailing lists for travel companies; getting videos on locations from the library—all of these can happen on any one day.

Want to lose fifty pounds? Begin with cutting out two slices of bread TODAY. Alternatively, one could say, "Let's get that into the New Year's resolutions." Gyms experience a surge of enrollments after New Year's and a drop in attendance by the end of January. So cut out the bread, and do not expect annual goals to substitute for daily goals set and kept.

Maintaining a bias for action coupled with keeping goals and daily monitoring works wonders for getting things done and maintaining movement toward some of those far-reaching goals. Consider the following:

- You cannot start doing something new any sooner than today.
- You can procrastinate and never get it done.
- Letting things slide often is the costliest decision one can make.

Does this mean that most of our big decisions were made quickly or with some extended help plan? No. Perhaps we might have wanted it to be that way, but such is not always the case. For example, we decided to relocate to Kansas City, which was not the center of activity in our fields of expertise. That decision came together just as Barbara was leaving government to either return to academic work or do something else. Monty was finishing law school and had no definite plans for what to do next. Possibilities existed for both of us but nothing conclusive. At the same time, Barbara's mother was living alone in Kansas City and wanted her to return, work nearby, and be there for her in person.

We had no firm plans for alternatives, so we said, yes, why not? We can live and work from there. This decision limited further options, but we were able to both search for opportunities and begin to sell our services as consultants. The consultant route flourished. It didn't turn into a growth business model, but it did lead us to do work that used our skills and met the needs of many clients.

In short, it was a personal consulting model, not one with a defined product that could be delegated to junior people or put into a computer to generate reports that we would sell. It was personal consulting and unique models designed for specific clients. It worked for us, and it worked for our clients. It was professionally satisfying but not the beginning of a company that could mass-produce anything. It was a model for an artist or public thinkers; it suited us perfectly but isn't a model for everyone to follow. We recommend it to those who wish to pursue creative ventures wherever they might lead without the rule of universities. Perhaps it could work with think tanks. We chose the path not often taken. It was a good life then and now in our active aging. Continuing to find creative ways to move forward, we rejoice in our choices.

Meditation and Mindfulness

In thinking about the uses and benefits of meditation and mindfulness, we considered discussing them in the psychology section. They are mental and physical, really whole body activities and often studied and recommended. Meditation also could have been covered in the spirituality area. Meditative practices and mindfulness are at the heart of many religious and spiritual activities.

We discuss mindfulness and meditation here because they are practices that have become tools of thinking that aid in calming an overactive mind. Mindfulness and acting in the present are, for us, mostly the same thing. Many of the meditative practices are essential elements in the crafting and methods of life designs. We not are living our lives as separate spheres of work and leisure, nor as work or spirituality, or as work or something else. To us, the life of the mind, body, and spirit are not separate. Our living of work/life was not different in nature from our living an active presence in retirement; they are merely ongoing expressions of our sense of the way a busy life unfolds in reality.

Meditation is the process of spending habitual time developing a quietness of mind, sometimes with a focus on God or a word or image one wishes to inculcate. In all practices, one becomes a calmer, stronger person. For us, meditation has evolved both as a form of worship and human self-improvement. Meditation and mindfulness are tools for making correct decisions. Meditation is useful for living in its many modes of expression—work, leisure, activities, or retirement. Being in touch with the core of life invigorates it all, not just some of it but all of it.

Meditation as a regular practice focuses attention on one's breath or a visual object or a silently spoken word or phrase. The goal of this activity is to become more sensitive to the inner working of one's mind. Over time, one becomes more adroit at living in the present moment and skillful in finding ways of relating with others. It is also true that the spiritually attuned person can use meditation to achieve higher levels of communication with a Higher Power. Dedicated religious people do maintain communication with a Higher Power through meditative practices. However, others use meditation to strengthen their skills in mindfulness and to live in the present moment without any reference to spirituality or religion.

A person who wants to meditate can set aside a specific time and a special place to sit quietly for a prescribed amount of time. During this time, the person can be quiet, perhaps focusing on breathing alone. The time can also be used to review the life goals and significant events occurring in one's life. Others may use it to condition thinking to achieve goals. For example, one can visualize being more fit, doing more exercise, or lifting weights.[17]In achieving overall wellness and fitness, meditation is used to support an active spiritual life and to engage in a very healthy and active aging life.

Meditation time can be about anything, including one's joys, sorrows, plans, dilemmas, and future goals in becoming kinder and more loving to others. Any meditator can do the same kinds of reflections on how to become a better person. One can also use the calming time to reflect on the day's events coming up and how to engage in them in

---

17   Today we think of meditation, visualization and mindfulness when working to condition our thinking. In Monty's early years he would be reading Norman Vincent Peal's writings or some other motivational book of the time. Positive psychology, positive thinking, affirmations of varying sorts seem to work. We believe that our thoughts do have an impact on our thinking, our mood and our actions. Have our successes in life been because of this kind of thinking? Or our failures due to neglect to develop more positive thoughts. Who really knows? We tend towards the positive and it is a force in our lives.

specific ways to carry out the kinds of actions needed to achieve one's health and life goals.

During meditation, a person strives to quiet the mind and body to be receptive to one's inner voice. For the religious practitioner, this is a time to listen to the sound of God speaking to you. For others, it may be a quieting of the mind to allow one to calm down to better focus one's attention. It may aid in calming the mind to focus on a particular problem or issue.

There are perhaps as many perceptions of what meditation is like as there are practitioners. However one goes into it, the outcome is likely to be more peace of mind. Through meditation, inner peace and a resolve to be fully aware of each moment become a habitual way of seeing the world and relating to its processes. It is a powerful way to ready oneself for the challenges of life.

Spending time each day in quiet meditation also helps a person grow in mindfulness in accomplishing essential tasks to be carried out each day. Bringing a sense of calm to a person's body and mind allows the individual to drop stress, irritability, and knowledge of being driven to the activities of living in a high-pressured society.

Being quiet and focused also permits the entire body to systematically carry out daily functions such as sleeping, eating, processing and eliminating nutrients. It also facilitates the normal bodily processes of sensing and responding to minor physical ailments in a quiet and more orderly way.

Daily meditation is a discipline that we find is useful in leading an active life. It usually demands time set aside at various periods throughout the day in a quiet setting where you can be involved entirely and free of all distraction. Do this daily. It is constructive to focus intent on specific behaviors one wishes to strengthen. Moreover, it can easily be the occasion for setting daily goals with action steps to be done that day. It is a powerful way to achieve successful change in one's life.

There is a strong relationship between meditation and mindfulness. Habitual meditation improves one's mindfulness capacity. When a person becomes more mindful, she knows what is happening "right here, right now" and accepts this reality while dealing constructively with the immediate situation calmly and positively. Such a person doesn't run away from a complicated human scenario but examines the entire situation being played out and deals calmly first with the important and then the less essential elements in the situation.

Growth in mindfulness capability is an essential outcome of successful meditation. It also assists a person in becoming more focused, sensitive to present realities, and calm amid the irregular ups and downs of dealing with the stress of real-life situations. In short, meditation trains us for mindfulness, thus meditators tend to be more mindful.

Mindfulness is being open and aware in the present moment, without criticism or mind wandering. Mindfulness gives a person additional energy to focus on the problems at hand and to constructively solve them.

A state of mindfulness permits opportunities for seeing and experiencing in the present moment broader aspects of life; i.e., beautiful sunsets, the quiet of walking in the woods, and the love expressed between members of a family.

While meditators can become more mindful, which, in turn, can improve decision-making, meditation should not be a cause of nor an excuse for procrastination. Not deciding can be the wrong decision.

No Decision *Is* a Decision

Delay is a choice. Delay caused by lack of proper information leads to another good lesson: if you don't know to move ahead with a final decision, start the research; build prototypes or mental models; or flesh out ideas about choices. Make each day count for progress in growing your ideal lifestyle. To decide where in the country we wanted to retire, we used three mental models to assist us: brainstorming; a SWOT (Strengths, Weaknesses, Opportunities, and Threats) analysis; and a Scenario Building Exercise.

Brainstorming

Deciding where we would live our retirement years was a significant decision, so we asked several people individually and in groups for their suggestions. Employing this method of soliciting different ideas was most helpful for us.

The brainstorming technique is easy to employ:

- All ideas are welcome.
- Write down the ideas so everyone can see them.
- No one is to criticize any idea.
- After the ideas are listed, the people involved in the process can discuss the options more freely.

Strengths, Weaknesses, Opportunities, and Threats Analysis

In discussing where to live, one inevitably begins to develop criteria about the personal strengths and weaknesses of each location. All kinds of reasons are behind the brainstormed list: low cost of living, great theater nearby, close to family, and so on. Our move from Washington, DC, to Kansas City was based more on a strong desire to put family issues above all else. It also came at a time when other choices were not uppermost in our minds. On the other hand, the last move from Washington, DC, came after months of sorting through options and the exploration of possibilities using most of our analytic techniques discussed here.

From the list of places that surfaced during the brainstorming session, we looked at the strengths, weaknesses, opportunities, and threats of each site and then applied a numerical code to the desirability of the place against our criteria for strengths and opportunities. To gain more information, we read about and discussed possible places with professional colleagues. We also visited locations, sometimes having clients in the area, to get a feel for them.

One retirement center on a university campus was attractive, but the university choice of sites was in more of a rural area and lacked the medical elements that we wanted. Another was near downtown and campus, but again, no major medical complex. Both were favorites of our ideation and mental modeling discussions, but we visited neither. A medical complex component held a strong pull for us.

To begin our sorting out places, we did a value analysis of the criteria that we were developing. As we discussed where to live, we identified the reasons for each location. Our rules were related to our list of desires and values for our retirement.

We wanted to stay reasonably close to a major university. Why? We thought we might do some teaching later, and we also desired the campus atmosphere. Our ties to health care led us to favor a research and teaching hospital nearby. If it had a program in health administration, that would offer some part-time teaching opportunities.

Active aging opportunities already were high on our list of attributes, so they made it onto a list. Hiking was part of that, so the idea of being near a protected forest or ocean kept coming up.

We put Chapel Hill, NC, at the top of the list, although locations in Arizona, Colorado, and California also were in contention. Chapel Hill's strengths included ties to both Duke University and the University of North Carolina and familiarity from having lived in Chapel Hill for several years. We both could do some teaching at two universities. We also had many friends in the area, and Monty has family in the Carolinas. Excellent medical care would have been available there, and ample work and leisure activities were all around. Chapel Hill would have placed us in a familiar setting. Chapel Hill had much of the pull of a homing instinct, the familiar, a family, the lure of good years past.

So we searched for a house, found one, and, after a first offer, we were about to make a counteroffer when it occurred to Monty that our desire for either mountains or the sea was not part of the package. However, one attraction of the house we were about to buy was its Southwestern attributes. It reminded him of Arizona. Arizona represented the pull of the frontier, the unexplored, another life experience. So the hunch to go to a new adventure was an intuitive leap, with the lure of new challenges and beauties to discover.

The decision completely changed our direction. We switched from going home to the familiar to entering a world new to both of us. It's an excellent example of how intuition, sensing, and feeling play essential roles in our lives. We can only imagine just how different life might have been if we had not listened to that "sense" of what to do.

We have no regrets about that choice. We now see it as inspired. We chose a learning opportunity over the comfort of the known. We opted for novelty over the known. We wanted an area where physical activity would be a top priority, not a place where intellectual pursuits would dominate and require repopulating our friendships. In short, we had ideas for the new life-plan model and chose locations in which we could flesh it all out. It was a gamble. We won but didn't know that this choice would demand a few years of effort to live out our dreams.

Two days later, we boarded a plane to scope out Phoenix and surrounding areas. Before we left, we had contacted a real estate agent in Tucson, who ultimately found the right place for us. It had almost everything on our list. The house we bought was a short walking distance into a national park wilderness area. All of the ideation, the searches, and the sorting-out process worked exceptionally well. We bought the new place and moved within two months of our epiphany.

Our active aging interest in the outdoors, fitness, and our only "sport"—walking—turned out to be an essential criterion. Arizona was high on our list, with wide-open spaces, clear night skies, and mountains in all directions. Adventure tugged harder than our more-conservative concerns for additional work in our chosen profession.

The "threat" component is a significant variable in the SWOT analysis. In retirement, we saw two considerable risks: exhaustion of resources or a debilitating illness. Right insurance and medical and support resources would be needed.

Another threat is the earning capacity of the person or couple. We both were prepared for multiple kinds of occupations with sufficient earning capacity for both, even if one was not working. That made savings and reserve contingencies possible. We both landed part-time work after "retirement," but when it became apparent that we could do without the pay and the work failed to meet our interest, we retired. However, we did not entirely withdraw all of our professional skills and attention.

Before the point of retirement, however, we asked a financial institution to do a thorough analysis of our situation. After completing that process, we learned that we could retire with confidence if our expenses stayed within our then-limits, and, if nothing catastrophic happened, we would have sufficient resources for long life when we retired. It also meant that we did not need more paying jobs to follow our life dreams of doing other things. That was comforting, but it was no excuse for not doing some of that financial planning sooner. We had the right attitudes about work and saving but neglected the monitoring of our finances and what that can do if and when adjustments are needed. To remedy that, we found skilled legal and financial consultants to keep us on the right track. With more considerable attention to this detail, we might not have tried out post-retirement, part-time jobs. However, like most such mistakes, one never really knows. The past is the past.

Scenario Building

In the first stages of our retirement journey, we found ourselves in a new state and city, in desert terrain with four acres of land abutting a National Park . . . all new experiences for us. We had reached the desert via intuition. Our more rational efforts to plan retirement occurred after being in our brand-new environment. Our history of life together included two university towns and three very large cities not in a desert next to a wilderness. So we began to spend time developing our personal goals as a couple for success in our new world. We had worked out our own life scenarios for our retirement years. Now we could try them on. Some fit, most did not.

A scenario is a well-thought-out plan for a major event, an important challenge, or a section of a person's life.

We spent intensive time in our first months in Tucson defining how we were going to begin to live our retirement. That was also a life design project, although at the time we did not call it by that name. As we've noted, getting to Tucson was more intuitive than rational, but now as we write about it, we are rationalizing how it all happened. Thinking, feeling often happens that way.

Our overarching goals remained mostly the same, but how they played out was determined by the environment of the desert, not a college town.

The essential goal areas we wanted to focus on were these:

- Learn the realities of living in the Sonoran Desert.
- Develop friendly relationships with our neighbors, even though all were in four-acre or larger plots.
- Continue our dedication to a healthy diet and outdoor exercise.

- Examine the access to comprehensive health services.
- Research opportunities for volunteering for community activities.
- Develop creative outlets in art, music, and the study of Native American culture.

From Brainstorming to Reality

The planning tools we used eventually turned into a decision. The turnabout from a university town in North Carolina to a desert city with acreage near a national park was a giant leap but not inconsistent with our main criteria. An old sheet of yellow paper held the list of our criteria and was last used before that decision point. It specified proximity to

- A good university for possible courses to teach.
- A well-developed airport for travel and consulting.
- Beautiful natural resources for outdoor recreation and walking.
- State-of-the-art medical care.
- Proximity to relatives.

Without using the thinking tools for problem identification and solving, and the weighing and sorting of most meaningful criteria, this critical decision might well have left us disappointed rather than elated with our choice.

Did we get it right? For fitness and regaining our health with exercise, healthful eating, and time outside with nature, we did. We also found a neighborhood where we really could have social contacts and build a new life. Ultimately, our decision to settle in Tucson was not ideal for any semi-retirement plan to return to lesser roles in health care. And family? Not close but a free-standing guest house was available for their use when they visited. Barbara has few even distant relatives, and Monty's sibling are deceased and his daughters living in noncontiguous states.

Ahead of us lay writing, art, and active living. We counted the positives to be much more critical than the paths not taken. We loved the ones we chose. Mistakes often are right decisions in hindsight.

Think and Plan for Active Aging

Before the actual doing of active aging, first think about it. Being alive and functioning means you already are active. However, if you want your long life to be the best it can be, plan to make it so. Don't neglect your feelings about things included in plans; they may well be the best indication of what will work for you. For example, our early plans suggested being close to nature and also in proximity to high tech medical care. Those two features are near polar opposites and rarely exist in close proximity. The early sites considered in Arizona were in the northern part of the state. By holding onto both criteria we found a medical school in southern Arizona adjacent to a national park, an ideal choice for us.

As the Star Trek Captain Kirk might say to the navigator, "Lay in a plan to get there, then turn to the engineer and say, MAKE IT SO!"

Keep in mind that because we also are our captain, planner, and an engineer, it's all up to us to do the work required.

There are many ways to achieve goals and, no doubt, other ways yet to be invented. Some might take a brisk walk, enjoy it, and make it a habit over time. Others might follow a passion for work that keeps them active without a specific plan; they just remain busy. Our pool maintenance man, for example, had been in the business for thirty-four years. He got into pool maintenance by helping a friend, and, after finding that being outside working on pools was so enjoyable, he started his own business.

Because there are many options to get involved in an exercise, the first step might be to examine a few possibilities. Our options were swimming, walking, yard work, gym membership, Tai Chi, and spinning. Each has tradeoffs. Consider walking:

Pros

- Free in the neighborhood and nearby park
- Requires only a good pair of shoes
- Many ways to do it each day

Cons

- Requires discipline to established routines
- Might need pricey fall-alert system to get help on back roads
- Wildlife in the area might be a danger

In the end, we combined neighborhood walking, parking lot excursions, and treadmills at the gyms. Tai Chi, yoga, and spinning became regular activities for several years. When our instructors left, we found ourselves adrift from these practices and fell back to hiking and a YMCA gym membership, where treadmills, weights, and machines were available.

How one develops good habits matters less than the fact of their development. Good habits are to be valued, whether learned naturally, or thought about and adopted according to a plan. For those like us whose work did not require much physical exercise, having a plan is helpful, and decision tools are useful in sorting things out before beginning a journey. After doing the research for this book and getting up to date on the latest ideas, Monty decided to get a trainer to check his style and recommend improvements.

Hit the Ground Running

We acted quickly on the decision to go to Arizona. After we arrived, we found ways to implement our physical fitness goals. Our general life plan unfolded more or less as we had envisioned, but those initial plans were only concepts and mental models. A four-plus-acre complete with 5,200-square-foot living space—a principal and guest house—was a challenge to furnish and learn to use.

One part of our plan worked from the outset: it took much active energy to keep the place going, and we got our ration of daily steps in part by walking 200 yards to the gate for the mail! The first neighbors we met lived three-quarters of a mile away—a long walk or a short ride. There was much to learn, but we knew the essential elements. It was a big challenge to learn how to use the space best. Later we refined the uses and spent heavily, making the place even more functional.

Was it easy to find new friends? Asking neighbors about cactus to avoid wasn't hard to do after finding oneself festooned by spines from a Cholla cactus. Just touching one of those prickly plants provided a strong incentive to reach out and ask for help. When the wind blew down a tree and your car was underneath, a neighbor with a fork-lift would be there to help. Help was always close by, and after a few incidents like this, we got to know the neighbors. People helping one another adds spice for social relations. Exchange occurs when people are in smaller groups where neighbor helping neighbor is the primary source of help.

As we became more involved in the Medical Reserve Corp and the broader community, our hiking and classes slowed. We lost some of the fitness we had gained through a more active focus just on ourselves. In the sixth year of our retired life in Tucson, Monty began work on a memoir. He started writing it on September 10, 2001. On the second day of writing, he watched TV pictures of planes flying into the World Trade Center in New York City! What might have been an autobiography became a combination of an autobiography and accounts of current events. New developments in science impact our behaviors.

Our volunteer activities were much different from the work we had done as consultants and educators. When volunteers do their jobs, the emergencies they help counter can be grueling and dangerous. But crises are few and infrequent, so we train. Our training required planning, coordinating, study, and travel. We took many courses and traveled to meetings as well as some weeklong programs. However, the demands on volunteers and the role we were expected to play were limited. For Monty, this was a setback. He volunteered to serve in AmeriCorps to get a Medical Reserve Corps established. He then recruited physicians and others to head it. Such professionals are essential to the design and functioning of medical care teams. However, those who typically employ and deploy AmeriCorps volunteers are accustomed to having young college-age people doing low-level assistant work. So when Monty began to contact leaders in the emergency response hierarchy in order to find the right fit for a reserve corps composed of professionals. His supervisor was startled at him going immediately to work on the agencies in charge. He viewed contact with them as his personal responsibility and immediately directed Monty not to talk with anyone such as the regional director of disaster response without him being present. That nullifying action made design work difficult so Monty spent much of his time studying disaster planning and relief efforts, time well spent but an impediment to doing the work he volunteered to do.

One of the ideas Monty developed was submitted for a national meeting in Washington, but the supervisor refused to allow Monty to use any duty time to attend. He felt Monty should scale down and serve as a call operator for people wanting to volunteer. This fraught relationship continued, so Monty went to the meeting in DC using his own funds and unpaid time. He took lots of courses online via the Federal Emergency Management Agency, got doctors recruited, and finished out his term of hours, mostly studying and learning about the way emergencies are managed—another aspect of his more general management skill set.

In spite of the narrow confines of that first job, the Medical Reserve CORPS was launched. Monty was then asked to serve on the Citizen Corp Council for Arizona (CCCA), and Barbara and he started the Community Emergency Response Team for our neighborhood. Monty chaired the CCCA for Arizona before just working our area. Within a couple of years, his passion for painting became a focus for his energies. He had turned a corner and was beginning a new chapter of life.

No Wasted Efforts

Things that initially seem a waste need not be so. We did meet and use the various learnings in strengthening our neighborhood and our survival and caregiving skills. Much of this knowledge is ours to use as we go on through life. Courses we took to become information officers in emergency work continue to inform our learning and interpretation of rules and edicts. We learned that what is provided for public consumption is information the agency (government or business or social) uses to drive behavior in a desired direction. This kind of understanding helps to sort the reasoning behind the messages sent. Unfortunately, it often leaves us skeptical when messaging comes from government bodies during hotly contested political campaigns.

Circumstances Can Intrude

In our consulting work and teaching, we stressed the need for continual mental modeling. Planning requires mental modeling, and then some of that thinking gets into formal and published plans. Published plans are the ones spoken of by generals and others as "the plan fails to be a reliable guide once the enemy is engaged." Once one begins to implement a plan, there is the reality of REALITY. It rarely is just what one was thinking. It is when one engages in building out their mental models that the value of those models is enhanced or dashed. Often, one already will have imagined what happens in real time and is surprised but partially prepared by having considered such options in the thought process.

As we aged, the property—two houses, studio spaces, offices for writing, and lots of space for guests—required too much work. What was a useful amount of space to keep us active, including stairs, became a burden rather than a benefit. The work, recreation, and playtime that we wanted and needed was eluding our grasp. What once was easy access to medical resources became more of a chore and less of a pleasure.

In short, we needed a new plan for active aging beyond eighty. Neither of us ever anticipated living much beyond our parents. Both fathers died in their mid-sixties, and both mothers died shortly after age eighty, although we were already retired when that happened.

Nearing eighty ourselves, we decided to plan for a retirement without the burdens of Spirit Base Camp. We had looked at options, and Kansas City remained a most likely fit for us. Our love of the desert and continuing good health kept this change process in low gear. However that love gave way to the judgment that we needed to move while still able to do it and to get settled before health issues hit.

Now in our mid-eighties, we are way beyond our planned-for life spans. Our current planning horizon allows for reaching one hundred, and we do not consider it likely. But it could happen. This life design for health project and book writing has made the longer life more likely and not less so. We have witnessed in ourselves changes predicted for those who engage in the active aging elements elaborated upon in these pages.

Over the years, we had participated in the planning and implementation of integrated health care systems, many of which either owned or operated Continuous Care Retirement Communities (CCRC), now called Life Planned Communities. We resumed an earlier planning approach by going over the list of places already considered. One or two were near Duke and UNC; one was in Tucson; and another, which we had not seen but knew about, was in Kansas City. It was near St. Luke's Health System, a former client, and less than a mile from Kansas University Medical Center. Moreover, all of this within a few minutes' drives to major cultural attractions. Even with all of these resources nearby, the most important resources include our learning from this research and writing AND the daily decisions to implement these ideals.

In some of our earliest planning notes, one criterion stood out—retiring where the family lived. Had we retired in the Carolinas, Monty's family would be nearby, or in Kansas City, Barbara's family would be nearby. So in our eighties, we followed through with this criterion, which meant that Barbara, after Monty's demise, would be near family. However, our thinking is less than perfect on those criteria. At our advanced age, few of Barbara's family are left to be near!

As we reflected on the difference between our thinking when we were younger than sixty-five versus at age eighty-plus, it became apparent to us that service proximity, especially medical service, was an important variable for our retirement. So we added a new criterion to replace our earlier concern for being in nature; we decided that proximity to all we might need and enjoy should be within a walk or easy drive or cab ride from our dwelling. To live actively and enjoy our primary life interests, it was clear to both of us that we were near the limit of our time in the desert. Since family support may not be readily available when needed, it is best to plan to be near other forms of support from service providers. While individual providers will change over time, institutional values are likely to remain.

Time for Change

Around 2012, it was only a matter of timing as to when we would move. Monty was getting signs that his heart needed close monitoring. Our choices of places quickly narrowed to Kansas City, where excellent medical resources were near at hand. Alternatively, we could stay in Tucson at a CCRC and continue to enjoy the desert. With this choice, the excellence of medical resources near a CCRC and the amenities of a larger city made Kansas City the logical choice. Institutional support was just a few minutes from a high-quality retirement center.

We had long known about and evaluated services in the locations under consideration and all were excellent, but Kansas City had the added advantage of being close to many of Barbara's old friends and her few relatives. We would also be living in the heart of the city, so we could explore more of our artistic interests in painting, theater, and the variety of creative arts that can be found only in large urban centers. We didn't need a new SWOT or other devices to narrow the choice. Over the years, we had effectively narrowed the field, making a final selection easy.

Living so far out from neighbors and medical services and without much human contact was excellent for our early explorations but much riskier as we could sense some decline

Barbara was already stressed with routine work at SBC. Monty's heart surgery required long drives at night and obtaining assistance from neighbors to care for him. Old age presages such declines and the need for readily available help. Our desert retreat was becoming more liability and less of an asset for great health. We had done all the planning, and so we were only making our final choices, talking it all over, and beginning to discuss with family and friends. When we made the formal move, we didn't need to do much except contact the community and make a trip to conclude a deal. Notably, we were prepared to buy into the retirement center even though we had never visited it. It fit our scenarios and if anything was missing, we felt competent to handle the challenge of the unknowns.

Our well-honed tools have made most of our decisions the right ones. That said, it would be best to remember that how well things work out depend heavily upon how one CHOOSES to view them. The night skies in the desert offered eternal beauty in our hearts, minds, and on canvas. In Kansas City, we live among the jewels of human-made art, music, entertainment, and science. Each has its beauty. The tools of our trade helped us to find these places, first in our minds then in our actions.

As this book draws to a close, we are at another crossroad. Should we move on to related publishing projects or spend energy to publish and share this work? Who knows just how this round of searching will go? There are pressures to go each direction, but time and energy resources are dwindling, thus harder choices will need to be made.

CHAPTER EIGHT (Q&A)

1.   Is that all of the major tools one needs?

Not by a long shot. There are probably as many ways of thinking about such issues as there are minds to define the problem. Each of us has ways and means we use to solve problems. When sitting near a computer, one of us will often search for keywords that come to mind. Usually, that delivers a host of questions. Sometimes we call a friend to discuss the problem. Someone with different training and experiences might take another pathway. For some, that might be utilizing the services of particular specialist. Our search is wide and loosely organized at the beginning, narrowing as reasonable scenarios come into mind.

2.   Are some aspects of problem-solving more important than others?

It is difficult sometimes to solve a problem as first framed. For instance, Monty was asked to put his paintings into a beauty shop. The shop was in a trendy area with lots of good energy around it. However, there was a sense that pictures priced higher than fifty dollars were too pricey. Well, that is about what it costs just for materials for an original painting. Usually, an agent gets 10 to 15 percent, the store receives 40 percent, and the artist about half. At $50, that would work out to a considerable loss. However if the store would use the paintings as decor and, say, either run a sale at $50 and maybe offer a drawing to win a free picture, the frame of reference for putting paintings in that store would shift. There would then be room for ways to compensate the artist while making new customers for the store. Reframing a scenario is often essential for problem-solving.

3. Does reframing a scenario change the problem or lead to another kind of problem?

In the case of the art example, reframing provides access to another whole set of problem-solving approaches. Monty had lots of graduate work in business and marketing, so he stopped thinking like a painter. The painter sees the art as needing a home and finding the right buyer. However, the marketer is looking for a match between a buyer and customer. In this case, the beauty operator would need to buy into a promotional concept and not see the paintings as a shelf product to sell directly. So, for Monty, the shift was into a very different way of thinking. If the beauty shop wants original art, they must essentially do the same thing. At this writing, the answer remains open. However, the marketing ideas will be used in other settings, so for this problem-solver, the situation is already a plus.

4. Are there other ways of reframing issues such as weight loss?

There are. Monty got some DNA testing and found that his weight is on average going to be above the norms for his height, so he always faces that heritable trait of needing to stabilize his weight above the norm. So he reframed the issue. Now he manages his weight 7 percent above the recommended standard and tries to keep it within 5 percent of that slightly elevated weight. That new norm is doable for him. It still requires watching things closely but not obsessing in attempting to reach a near impossible goal.

5. Much of this book is about retirement. Were there any major books you used to guide your thinking about retirement?

Yes and No must be the answer here. In our professional work we advised and help design health system who serve the sick and injured. Many of our clients also owned and operated retirement facilities. So we knew a lot about the service sector and what it has to offer. Our work and living in and around educational institutions informed our judgment about places to live at different ages. Our daily reading provided lots of information about financial and work affairs, retirement included. No doubt we scanned many stories about retirement but we bought no books on the subject. It would be helpful to read such book and articles. All of the methods used here can help but for each element of ones plan research will be required. Any given passion may well direct ones attention to other resources.

CHAPTER NINE

Implications for Individuals, Providers, and Policy

Life is sweet by itself, a feast rarely a famine
Join in the fun, Live fully today; tomorrow never comes
Live, dance, hold hands
Celebrate life at its fullest
Come, let's howl at the moon

Rooted in our mind's knowing lies the central truth:
The wisdom of the body holds the key to our health
Apply the magic of work and play
Nourish on fiber, whole plants, & fruit
Toss the sugar, flour, & manufactured foods
Revive the feast and famine cycles
Remember Nature, our prime physician

Reject the dependency of easy and free
Take the challenging road
Stand on your own,
Balance your Life
Live active and free

Writing Our Final Chapter

Our friend Douglas Green suggested the title for this chapter. It does signal an end to this particular writing. However, our philosophy is to live actively until the end of life. As Doug noted, Bob Dylan says, "He not busy being born is busy dying." We are busy learning new things, exploring life, and continuing to write and be active. Life is for the living; dying comes soon enough and will offer its lessons. Now is time for living. Each day is like a new birth; all of life is in front, the past is past, today is for living fully.

This book profiles our life together after retiring in 1995. Our active aging journey is about living positively in today's environment with its existing food production system, its medical systems, and our life circumstances. Of course, we were working on these ideas long before 1995. Moreover, we will be writing after this book is complete. We are creating the lifestyle best suited to our age and circumstances. In doing so, we shall also be commenting upon the ideas that seem pertinent to share with others, including our fellow professionals now running the health care systems and guiding national policy.

Many factors go into active living. Our history in health care is a significant factor in adding to our knowledge of the issues of healthy lifestyles, the underpinning of wellness for active aging. But in living out these years, much that we have learned applies to most people. Among the most critical factors we profiled were ideals we would like to attain in the broad areas of our life. These include:

- Good eating habits
- Regular physical exercise
- Regular intellectual exercise
- Strong self-concept
- Growth in spiritual development
- Participation in healthy social networks

Concurrent with living and redesigning our life style while writing this story, we are settling in at Bishop Spencer Place (BSP), a Continuing Care Retirement Community (CCRC) affiliated with Saint Luke's Health System in Kansas City, Missouri. So, as we compose the story of our active aging adventures, we are learning to live in a retirement community attached to an extensive health care system that includes sixteen hospitals and campuses across the Kansas City region. This system of services also offers home and hospice care, behavioral health care, and dozens of physician practices. In addition, we are only one mile from the Kansas University Medical Center, a complex system of services that complement those available within the BSP complex.

Nestled here among the kinds of institutions that we studied and worked with during our professional lives, we are daily alerted to ways in which they might perform to serve us and others better. So, embedded here are ideas for active agers and healthcare institutions for serving our community.

As a result of these resource-rich affiliations, we find ourselves in a sophisticated organizational culture whose mandate is primarily to serve the acute and chronic care of a large population base. Looking back at our decision to come to this particular retirement community, we remain impressed with the diversity and complexity of this specific environment.

As we contemplate the recommendations about active aging for individuals, institutions, professionals, and public policy, we focus primarily upon things that can be done by ordinary people within the context of existing health care systems. Professionals—through direct advice and publications—advise on our choices, educate us on food, and counsel us on lowering stress and getting a good night of sleep. However, it is the individual, it is we who must learn what works for us, establish the right habits, select healthy foods, exercise, and—with our companions—lead an active life.

In this book, we summarize our two-year examination of the meaning of Active Aging for two people who committed to being role models for healthy lifestyles. In Tucson, we developed themes of eating right, moving, engaging in complex thinking, and growing in self-awareness and spiritual development. Also, we connected with many people and groups for fun and community service.

Now we live inside a complex organizational environment dedicated to maintaining and restoring health to a large population base. As we look at the possibilities before us, we are processing all we have learned to this point. We have laid out the barebones schema of critical features for following a healthy lifestyle as a person ages. The working definition of Active Aging that we test against new knowledge and recent experiences is:

Active Aging is a daily process of choosing to optimize opportunities to improve your health and the quality of life.

Applying this definition to the essential activities of Active Aging is a challenging task. The preceding chapters of this book lay out the search for answers and our uses of what we found. Here we review the main points and offer suggestions for how individuals, institutions, and public policy can be improved to serve us and others to help us with the task of living an active life. The exposition of our story and what we have examined along the way is the basis for the suggestions and recommendations that follow.

Eat Right

Professionals and scientists study food choices and their use in curing disease and staying healthy. Doing this brings exercise and improving social relations into the professional domain. When cures or benefits are found, then reimbursable programs can be offered to cure or mitigate diseases. As of now, this is a goal for most research efforts. However, at this time, the primary person responsible for one's health is oneself. Gaining knowledge is abetted by professionals and education, but the doing of the things required for good health remains with the individual. Each of us chooses daily and acts on those choices.

We are aware of the many things that can go wrong in farming, food manufacturing, environmental adjustments, and such that could jeopardize human health. Science opens our eyes to the use of food, lifestyle, and related issues to improve health and prevention before medicines can become useful in managing a disease process. The change to more personal responsibility and the use of fitness and food as a drug will occur. However, the vast array of interest devoted to the status quo carries the day on national policy, and that policy tends to favor cures by physical intervention and single medicines to reduce the problems presented by chronic diseases. Many of these medicines are helpful and complement a healthy lifestyle. However, it is not unusual that an active lifestyle can reduce the need for intensive medical regimens, so care needs to be taken to monitor the issues involved and change course when it is prudent to do so.

The solutions to the issues of social determinants such as income, social status, education, and literacy lie outside the usual domain of medical services. However, the knowledge needed to aid individuals to solve these issues does exist inside the medical care system. Thus, professionals and institutions should assist in their resolution. Every encounter with a patient is an opportunity to educate. When patients are hospitalized for countless hours of inactivity, that is the time for education to improve the patient's self-help capabilities. Opportunities such as these are too often overlooked when they don't represent evident revenue generation. And, we might add, no one in particular is in charge of strengthening the patient's self-help capabilities. As it becomes apparent that lifestyle is an essential determinate of health outcomes,

more professionals will find ways to develop and market assistive services using coaching and counseling techniques.

Business Decisions Impact Food Choices

Advertising and availability shape our choices. In the absence of positive advocates for healthy habits, most will miss the toxic implications
of choosing the highly visible and delectable sugar/fat/salt bomb. It is
never easy to overcome the daily cues that often bode ill for our good
health. We fall prey to temptation, to our detriment. However, it is
within the power of each of us to overcome, however slowly, at whatever
age. Our bodies, our natural systems, work endlessly to keep us going,
and it is often only after years of poor choices that our body systems fail.

Individuals face choices throughout the day. Those choices, for
good or ill, shape our health in ways that are opaque to most of us.
Science reveals more each day. Our attention here is a distillation of our
understanding of the best evidence and most useful advice at this time
in history.

Geriatric institutions should focus on a high level of wellness for
all residents. Some do. Others serve great food with love while leaving
aside healthy choices that improve health at any age. Sweeteners are an
example: Stevia is generally regarded as a safe sweeter, while many of
sweeteners chemically produced in the early shifts away from cane and
beet sugar get negative reviews. Those artificial sweeteners continue
to dominate the table, however. The excuse for this? Customers want
them. Does anyone accept the role? Surely professionals should do it,
and insurers should cover it.

Institutions face many choices. We assume that nursing homes,
continuing care retirement communities, and other services for the
aging population have expertise in the organization to make excellent
choices. We recognize that they make choices within the context of
existing knowledge, especially government guidelines and consumer

preferences. If more customers seek better opportunities for high-level wellness, those who catch this trend will be the ones getting the most customers.

For health care professionals to choose correctly, they must know the facts of current consumption patterns for the people they serve. Unfortunately, from a wellness perspective, those existing patterns are shaped by the dominant culture. Sugar, fat, and salt dominate the food system. The idea of retiring to leisure and being served after the young age of sixty-five or sooner contributes to becoming less active, not more active as good health might dictate.

Too much sugar, fat, and salt in the typical American Diet is at the heart of the obesity, diabetic, heart, and dementia epidemics. The nature of the food we consume is a direct causal factor for many of these issues. The social factors and our individual choices and habits, most within our control, are at the heart of what can be addressed to improve our health.

Over the years, we have tried every major diet fad. In our experience: *all diets succeed and all diets fail!* Our sense of diet approaches is that the approach used might need to be tailored to each individual's unique needs. At this point, what we need in our lives is different from what we sought in earlier times. Sometimes the advice from experts, the science community itself, changes our direction. Finding a balance of healthy foods is hard. The airwaves convey many contradictory messages, such as low carb, high carb; or, low fat, high fats.

The messages we receive about eating often carry the phony idea that we need three square meals per day and snacks to thrive. There is no truth to that assertion. Fasting daily for twelve to twenty-four hours has better science and common sense to back it up. Fasting works.

There are many technical reasons given for fasting. The first one, which appealed to us, is the fact that fasting is done by many in the Mediterranean region so famous for its dietary habits. Most recommendations for following this general diet of olive oil, red wine, and good fellowship leave out the fact that religions of the region had many feast and famine days. For many areas, fasting is a way of life.

When fasting, after the first few days of acclimating to the change in nutrition intake, the urgency for eating—especially snacks—disappears. We haven't tried all of the fasting methods, but skipping one meal and snacks came first. Then we tried eating within a few-hours window, say four to seven hours, which worked well. Our reading about and trying different approaches remains an ongoing exploration.

Move

We need strength, flexibility, and stamina. Moving our bodies is an active catalyst for our circulatory systems. Moving one's body affects the main muscle groups: lower body, upper body, and abdominal area (referred to as "core"). Every type of exercise impacts the brain. However, we need more than physical exercise, puzzles, reading, and study for the brain. We also need laughter, surprise, and adventure to supplement pumping iron, swimming, and other activities.

Individuals are often guilty of neglecting their power to act in their own best interest. At a new exercise class one day, the instructor was ten minutes late. One member said, "Let's begin and do the work. Another vocal member said, "No way. I am not doing anything I don't have to do." This was, in essence, an excellent example of our current health care dilemma. Far too few people are willing to do what only they can do to stay fit by moving their body with regular exercise periods each day.

Public policy tends to mirror the interests of the dominant institutions and interest groups. We are aware that our health insurance programs are tailored to spend on diseases that our institutions and professions diagnosis and treat. There is scant attention, beyond mere words, paid to interventions that might prevent or reverse essential disease processes. In our pre-retirement research, a leader of a national organization noted that they were interested in active aging. However, their programs focus on the same issues as the medical establishment targets. Their lobbying parallels that of those who must protect the status quo. The inference we took from this encounter was that the establishment wanted to claim the territory but keep the existing programs out front of their work. This phenomenon seems universal. Who wants competitors to take their customers or money away from established interests?

Again, we do not attempt to change those significant forces, but there are still adjustments that would support active aging for those who seek to maintain their good health until the end of their life span. Addressing those factors is our modest goal here. Health span is very much the dominant factor in life span, and life span, in turn, is dictated by what individuals can do to improve their health daily.

There are many choices open to individuals within the more general goals of existing systems. So we suggest that for those who choose to make an effort at optimal health, professionals should provide guidance for their journey. At the first encounter with a patient whose A1c levels approach pre-diabetes levels, for instance, health care professionals should first urge consideration of lifestyle changes, not drugs, to reverse the path toward diabetes. In the same vein, when a patient is in the hospital with a lifestyle issue such as obesity, provide some coaching to urge them to take steps to change. Nudge whenever an opportunity arises to move more of us toward wellness and away from disease.

For many life-enhancing needs, the temptation to advise is contained in one word: MOVE! However, to make movement a daily habit that remains uppermost in one's mind requires thinking and intentionality. Health professionals, especially physicians, are the most authoritative ones to provide this advice. More could be done. For example, at a recent meeting someone noted that one hospital in our region is actually providing some education to patients while in the hospital recovering from surgery. The education is about diet and fitness to prevent future problems. This should probably be standard practice everywhere. Professionals have the knowledge required; patients need it; and, while recovering from a recent failure might be the best time to provide that knowledge to get the behavior changes needed to prevent future failures.

For individuals, thinking about what one must do daily is key to success in any endeavor. Every day, it is essential to connect one's primary life goals into the context of what is possible today, in the present moment. It is insufficient, even self-deception, to imagine that forming a grandiose goal can work magic in and of itself. One needs to take that grand goal into the present and ask, "What can we do today to further that goal?"

Walking is one of the most straightforward and quickly done exercises. The new devices to monitor steps taken come with the advice to do ten thousand steps a day. In this age of suburbs and personal cars, everything is generally within easy walking from one's car, so getting enough exercise through walking requires planning and scheduling time to do it.

In our retirement community, walking is something to plan and elect to do. Since elevators reduce the need to climb stairs, for instance, even that minor workout becomes a conscious choice. Establishing a routine of movement needs to be planned. Bye-bye long sitting bout; hello movement whenever possible!

It is good to remember that regular physical activity helps a person

- Control weight
- Lower the risk of heart disease
- Lower the risk of type-2 diabetes
- Strengthen bones and muscles
- Improve mental health

Think

To survive in today's complicated society, we need to use our minds to solve problems, be creative, learn new subjects, guide our decisions, and make a contribution to the world around us.

Another reason to keep the brain active is to combat dementia and the possibility of Alzheimer's disease. Research dealing with this formidable health care challenge abounds. Without our mental abilities, much else in daily living becomes problematic.

There are many ways to stimulate brain health; exercise, nutrition, challenging activities. So we need to know the kinds of exercises that will help keep the brain active. Also, what types of foods should be on our plate or planted in the garden or ordered in the restaurant? We do many things to stimulate our brains. Exercise gets the blood flow going for our voracious reading habits. We also write, paint, and engage in discussions with friends. Other suggestions for brain health include:

- Concentrate on a healthy diet.
- Sleep eight or so hours every night. Sleep is essential. Naps are good.
- Listen to music. Music has positive impacts on the brain.
- Make it a habit to learn something new
- Write. Writing improves memory and thinking.

Strong Self-Concept

In searching for maturity, a person strives to be reliable and secure in knowing and accepting who they are as a person. They do this through the cultivation of these essential traits:

- Know their strengths and weaknesses.
- Focus on showing respect in relationships.
- Carry out daily activities with minimal stress.
- Confront new challenges.
- Accept outcomes without controlling.
- Exhibit serenity and a keen focus on life goals.
- Show people respect.
- Engage in creative pursuits.

Spiritual Development

Spirituality cuts to the core of who we are and what we hope to become as we relate to a God anchor in our lives. A person's relationship with God is individual, sacred, and often attached to a church structure. Spirituality motivates us at the deepest levels of our being.

People advanced in spiritual development manifest these characteristics. They:

- Live in the present and trust in God for all of life's events.
- Use meditative practices and grow in mindfulness.
- Routinely attend church functions.
- Read spiritual writings.
- Show respect and care for other people.
- Manifest ethical conduct in all their dealings.
- Align with like-minded people.

By singling out these attributes, we stress that the dimensions of spiritual and religious domains are of profound importance to humankind. The depth of these domains and their ultimate import is opaque to most of us most of the time but often sought after by reason and faith. The dimensions discussed here are a means to an end goal of connecting to God.

In the spiritual life, connection to a higher power facilitates meditation and mindfulness. As we engage in a deep relationship with God, we are drawn to quiet periods throughout the day to draw our attention to pondering the essential truths of a spiritual life. This process of being calm and turning our attention to our thoughts brings peace. In addition, routinely quieting the mind and focusing on profound truths becomes an antidote to stress; when someone is distracted and under stress, taking the time out for a walk in nature and stopping to smell the roses can be the perfect cure for the restless and anxious mind and body.

Connect

People dedicated to Active Aging are committed to having healthy and positive relationships with family, friends, and work colleagues. Life experience suggests that people who maintain social connections and cultivate good friendships have high self-esteem. Also, they have greater sensitivity for others and manifest positive human interactions.

On the flip side, experience shows that people disconnected from others lose incentives for living. As a result, they tend to more easily become depressed, pull away from stable human interactions, and consider ending their lives.

Those who stay busy with exciting endeavors, maintain social connections, and cultivate good friendships manifest high self-esteem, have greater empathy for others, and demonstrate more positive human interactions. Ideas for staying connected include:

- Planning and implementing inclusive social events,
- Attending classes to learn new skills,
- Broadening one's outlook on life through meeting new people,
- Developing an artistic outlet such as painting,
- Traveling to different cities and countries,
- Volunteering for community activities.

The bottom line in connecting with others is that the process of associating with other people helps a person reduce stress in their life. A successful strategy for doing this is to find those who can lend an ear when you are a bit down or having trouble in some aspect of your life. The best way to do this well is to be there for others in their time of need. While giving should be unconditional and without thought of reward for it, the truth is that things that go around tend to come around. The act of giving is a blessing to those who serve as much as a gift to others.

Staying in touch with family is an essential aging strategy. Being connected to family is a critical element in personal emotional stability for the individual and other family members. It is necessary for an older family member to show extra support for the young members. They face the challenges of growing up in a chaotic world, finding the right educational arrangements, and starting their own families. The quiet, stable influence of a family elder does wonders for those finding their way in a less than a peaceful world.

Many consider loneliness one of the biggest health problems of today. Having a stable family life as one grows older is a hallmark of emotional strength and a deterrent to going it alone.

Besides our family, we chose others to share our lives. In this sharing, Active Agers work on all of their health-focused strategies as they socialize. They know if they hang out with drug and alcohol users, they risk addiction issues. If they have a weight problem, they skip the happy hour with those who gravitate to fat/sugar/salty pastries and fried foods. They also choose not to compromise their professional role responsibilities in inappropriate social activities.

The bottom line in connecting with others is that we are social beings who depend on others throughout life in our family, work, neighborhood, civic, and religious endeavors. The Active Ager recognizes this and assumes leadership in connecting with others as they build strong ties to people with compatible values and life goals. Reaching out to others is one of the essential standards for being a high-performing person.

Future Impact

Between the two of us, we have one hundred years of work experience in health care and about fifty years of retirement; our thinking about and working on issues of active aging spans forty calendar years.

Barbara worked the clinical end of health care in nursing and later in management while Monty worked in labor relations in his early health care career and the management and organization of large-scale systems of services, collaboratives, and mergers. Both of us spent time studying public health with a focus on health policy and health system design. Our work dealt extensively with sharing what we learned via teaching and publishing. As researchers, academics, and consultants, we have been involved in a wide range of service designs and problem-solving.

Here, our intent is not to present a particular design or advocate a specific approach to problems but to present our desires for our needs and what we perceive to be the hallmarks of people who seek high-level wellness and a health span that equals their life span. We are convinced that the evidence of our research points to active aging as a solution to healthier lives and longer lives. We have sought this for ourselves but do not hold out out limited successes as role models. Each must follow their own path. We share our experience to aid in that endeavor.

We believe that each person is the primary architect of their lifestyle and choices. Thus, what *we* do for ourselves matters most. We are not victims of some lousy agricultural policy or of doctors who do good work treating us when broken but do not have answers for staying well.

What Do We Need from Institutions and Professionals?

The first thing we need is for the hospital, CCRC, or health care professional to recognize that what we need most is knowledge and motivation to do what will keep us well. Having said that, we are aware that few come to you asking for this recognition or service. Most encounters occur when people are ill or confused and need help. The health care system is loaded with the knowledge and skills to fix a single malady, alleviate pain, and manage the ills that bedevil people who have lost their well state of being.

Until now, medical practitioners and institutions have worked well to fix us in diagnosing our problems and to repair and maintain our lives during chronic illnesses. Moreover, they care for us as we become infirm. However fantastic that service is, it is not a substitute for a wellness orientation to living. The outstanding medical and caring industry fixes things and cares for our ills and needs as we become more dependent on others to maintain life. However, most chronic diseases require great independent action by the individual to mitigate against worse outcomes, to reverse, or, better yet, to prevent the disease. The massive failure of health policy gives too little recognition to this fundamental fact:

Individuals must do their part or we cannot solve the access and cost issues related to human health.

When we recently asked a physician, "Why don't you start your pre-diabetic patients on diet and fitness regimens to reduce diabetic tendencies or to reverse the disease?" she said, "Most do not come to me until it is too late." Our thoughts here apply to the first contact with a patient, during their treatment, and at discharge: there are lifestyle modifications that can help to prevent or reverse diabetes II. Can you help clients to find those interventions that work?

Can Healthcare Institutions Support Active Aging?

Here, our comments are more speculative about what the nursing home, the retirement community, senior housing, and others who serve those on an aging pathway mostly beyond the age of fifty can contribute. Why is this more speculative? In large part because we have not experienced many of the settings about which we know just a little bit, nor have we validated ideas that we have gained from investigating different approaches. So, at this point, we caution the reader to reflect with us and consider what might work in your situation. Consider any recommendations or suggestions here as informed speculation, perhaps worthy of an experiment but not to be understood as a proven dictum.

In recruiting future customers, consider whether you wish to attract clients dedicated to active aging as a group. To illustrate what we think will attract those seeking a high level of wellness, we suggest attention to

- Physical activity
- Mental activity
- High-quality whole foods
- Socialization
- Spiritual support
- Continuing education and mental stimulation

We think that many who seek to align their health span with their life span will emphasize these attributes and that institutions would be wise to cater to that desire. However, it is equally evident that there is a widespread belief that retirement is for more sedentary pursuits.

For the active ager, a visit to the gym and swimming facility would be in order. For those seeking a more sedentary lifestyle, the theater for movies, or a lunch or dinner with the most exquisite steak and lobster dinner with pie and ice cream for dessert might work better. Such a meal we might enjoy, but we would be turned off by its lack of sensitivity to healthier food choices. For others, it might be perfect.

One thing that might work well for both the more active and the more sedentary groups is to pay more attention to the sourcing of foods. This has become popular as a lure for customers. Many restaurants now source their ingredients from local organic farms. Diet and eating healthy require dropping the regular saturated fat, sugar, and salt concoctions. We recognize that may not be the case for those seeking a retirement of leisure and good home cooking with traditional ingredients. No doubt catering to a variety will be the course taken by most institutions.

Over time, even residents (patients, customers) who come seeking leisure might be converted to active agers when they see the energy and fitness associated with a different, more active regimen. Our recommendation is to meet your residents where they are but offer regimens that ultimately attract people to healthier lifestyles. It is to the institution's benefit to have more self-sufficient residents than those who require excessive attention and care.

Hospitals and physicians have other issues to resolve. At the outset of an encounter with a patient, it is helpful for that patient to provide an explanation of the problem(s) needing diagnosis. The provider can use the patients input and clinical data to provide a medical diagnosis. The choices we face with different treatment options, and what we can do about our condition(s) depends on judgements both patient and provider must make in concert. Whenever possible, opportunities to include are those that require the least intervention and the most involvement and responsibility of the patient. High-level wellness practitioners take responsibility for their health and insist on being an active player with caregivers in goal setting, treatment choices, and solutions.

So, our crucial piece of advice is that your assessments and prescriptions consider us to be the prime architect of our health. We will make mistakes, and not every recommendation will work. We don't expect perfection, but we do want engagement and for you to try first to help us correct things we do that aren't working.

In general, we prefer lifestyle interventions as a first-level approach rather than surgery or chemotherapy. Many methods might work before the higher-risk interventional approaches are necessary.

Public Policy

Public policy and insurers policy are close to the same in this section because Medicare is the driving force behind what is most likely to be covered and what treatments are to be reimbursed. Private health insurers tend to follow those parameters laid down by Medicare. Medicaid covers those who have insufficient resources to cover their needs for medical care. And Medicaid also tends to be the payer offering the least for most of the services.

Since individuals make the first decisions to seek medical services, they should be more involved in decisions and financial implications. One of the early examples of how an individual can lower cost by choices made can be illustrated here with an example. Moles on the skin can be cancerous or not. How individuals treat them can vary. A Band-Aid on an inflamed mole may or may not clear up the issue; is the inflammation from friction or an underlying cause? If one presents a mole to a family physician, the physician will likely try the Band-Aid treatment first for $50. Alternatively, the patient can try the Band-Aid first for $.05. Or, as one of us did, we can go to a cancer specialist and get a biopsy for $400. Insurance paid for the most expensive. Health Savings Account holders would choose the $.05 treatment first. Having great insurance and no major out-of-pocket cost, we made a wasteful decision. Would more upfront cost have changed that decision? Perhaps.

Next, as insurers do for safe driving and nonsmoking reductions, they should design their programs to encourage active aging lifestyle practices. If there is a proven method for reversing diabetes or heart disease, use it before interventionist methods. Some rehabilitation methods could be stronger, and more at-home coaching might be added. The field cries out for innovations in these types of issues.

When Canada first passed its national medical care program, a percentage of national health expenditure was devoted to building facilities and pathways for more exercise. We need highway and public transportation funding to be tied to means for encouraging more walking and fitness regimens.

On the nutrition front, we need a revolution. Medical education should include more about food as medicine. When agencies approve chemicals used in food production, the impacts on human health need more attention. Fasting and fewer/lower-calorie meals need to be encouraged.

The issue of panels to offer guidance for the department has much to be corrected. It is too easy for the insiders who favor medicine or surgery to dominate policy while those with lifestyle modification approaches are left out.

We have no reliable way to prevent this. Expertise has a leading role, but experts need challenges to their methods and outcomes. We can only add, please keep in mind that the human body comes with its mechanisms for staying healthy. First, do no harm.

CHAPTER NINE (Q&A)

1. **Do you have any regrets now about retiring in your early sixties?**

We do have reflections on that as an issue. It was not our intention to retire, and, in fact, we haven't really done so, although we are ready for another transition. At our current age, we rarely work for money. However, our study and leisure interests are costly and sometimes produce income. As is often noted, the expectation that one would to retire at such an early age was in the original Social Security planning. Retirement on Social Security would to come after many would have died, thus allowing social security to remain solvent. However, life extension into the late seventies is more the norm now, thus way to early for active agers to quit their working lives.

We both sought new professional employment directions, but they proved unsatisfactory. We earned appropriate salaries for our post-retirement professional work. Then our interest shifted, turning to more reflective writing, poetry, and a memoir begun at another historical pivot point—the attacks on the Pentagon and World Trade Center towers. After that, our professional skills were fully utilized in volunteer work until we were in our mid-seventies. After those volunteer post, personal hobbies became our forte. Barbara worked on art, biography, and culinary skills while Monty pursued acrylic painting on canvas and writing poetry.

In one of our post-"retirement" jobs, Monty served for a year in AmeriCorps, a low-paid volunteer type of work but with a commitment to work a certain number of hours. The work was professional in nature, but the position required minimal skills. The work needed for professional skills was easily done, short-lived, and left plenty of time for more study of emergency management—a related professional occupational arena, another opportunity to learn.

2. So, do you not consider what you are describing as retiring from professional work?

That is a fair question. Initially it was a mixture of both. We used our professional skills to continue our volunteer work, although it is rare for organizations to want volunteers doing what paid staff does. Our writing skills were directed more at personal projects rather than paid work for others. So this was a type of retirement that is a crossover transformation into another profession but these roles were unpaid or underpaid. Past writing rarely paid the bills; it did lead to paid work. As this volume is being completed, two others are in the works. Now the work is more a labor of love, rather than a breadwinner activity,

Life is for living, and this "work" is also our pleasure. In many ways, our life's work has always been related to our basic sense of purpose which was and still is to search for ways to improve health for people. Sometimes others pay for the work we do, but whether or not we get paid, the work continues. However, given its deep meaning for us, the pay is mostly to meet our needs for resources to live and cover some of the expenses for the work we continue to do.

3. This book seems to be a hybrid—part professional, and part diary and autobiography. Why did we wait so long to write it?

We rejected writing the book before walking the walk, living the experiences we thought would work but had not been tried. After having done that, we had thoughts about a couple different directions to take the book: We could have used direct quotes and issues being debated to illustrate the things we found. Or we could have, as we did, try some or most of the jobs recommended and discuss them mainly in the context of our experience and judgment. So we chose to follow our earlier decision—write about it after living it all.

There was one consistent issue throughout: because everyone's wellness journey is so different, much needs to be tailored to individuals. So, go out and read and do the things that work for you. Some of the books we found most useful are in an appendix.

4. **Still, this chapter dealing with advice for others seems like a bit of an urge to go back to the consulting work and get things right. Any truth to that?**

There is an urge to get our professional colleagues tuned into a few big ideas here. We know that individuals can—indeed, it is essential—make a positive difference in prevention, remission, and management of disease processes. Yet, this gets almost no attention. We knew this fifty years ago and often urged it. Still, those with the knowledge have found no way to bridge the gap between those who know and those who need to know. This is a costly gap; it causes endless suffering and burdens our economic system. By some estimates, if current trends continue, health care cost will take the entire federal budget.

Our contribution to reducing health care cost is this book. And our long lives for an extra decade or so will be proof enough of our thesis. Perhaps after another one hundred years, Monty's art will sell for enough money to support a cadre of coaches to promote Active Aging and wellness.

5. **As you contemplate the reading and research on these topics, where do you think you will go for more significant insights?**

Nutrition and eating remain high on our list. Many issues remain unsettled in that arena. Also, research on chronic diseases often points to changes in nutrition and eating habits to find ways to avoid illness or cure it. Few existing medical treatments can do this. Besides, if one seeks prevention strategies to cure or prevent disease conditions, taming eating habits is an excellent way to go.

Habits are difficult to change, though, so we have entertained having more fitness coaches. But the cost of care skyrockets if someone needs around-the-clock care or monitoring. For that, we consider the Alcoholic Anonymous (AA) model of volunteers.

In researching the AA model, we found some other connections. One was the centrality of members admitting the need for a superior being to influence one's behavior. And it turns out that the founder of AA had evolved this model after having used psychedelics that expanded his own awareness of the direction to take in his work.[18]

So we will continue to explore research that illuminates the mind-body or mind-consciousness connections and thought on related subjects.

6. **As you reflect on the factors noted in this volume, do they come together in a coherent way for you?**

---

18 Mr. Pollan mentions this in his book. Michael Polllan,*How to Change Your Mind: What the New Science of Psychedelics Teaches Us About Consciousness, Dying, Addiction, Depression, and Transcendence* Kindle Edition. We are great admirers of AA and its use of volunteers, addicts, who help one another. This idea is effective and could be further expanded perhaps using coaches in some realms of fitness and eating needs. Patients who have success in changing their lives are a good pool of potential health coaches.

Actually there are themes that come together in coherent ways. We tend to operate on a biological level looking at the work through lenses that isolate systems and categories. Much of science reaches into great depths to isolate cause and effect. The medical models, which have been the core of our education and work, operate this way. Our factors here are extrapolations from what is a holistic reality. In reality our so-called systems are fully connected and interact in ways beyond our imagination. But in our writing and meditations about this work, we can discern much of the factors and the exchanges among them. A spiritual moment may be the predecessor to a habit change just as a change in pills or food can trigger feelings that lead to changes in other activities such as sleeping habits.

7. Is there any area not covered here in depth that deserves greater attention?

There is one issue lurking behind this entire discussion, and that is the question related to brain, mind, and consciousness. Are we merely matter? Or, are we an energy matrix in a larger field that connects with other fields, all within processes that we now think of as the universe(s), and sometimes call the All? Or, as most religions posit, are we created in an image by God and life in a manner ordained by God? Here we are off and running, exploring the writings of others, our own prayers and meditations, and more.

CHAPTER TEN

Facing the Journey-Life Begins and Ends

The early stages are set by others
Later, we chose, we begin
Often the process repeats,
We learn, we grow
We earn, we save
We prepare . . . or not

There is time when work recedes
Some work on their business
Others continue a career, or a hobby
Some lie around and watch
Life goes toward sunset.
Fit is better than not
Healthy is better than creeping along

Life is movement, engagement
Life loves company
Life is work, play, and more
Life thrives on variety and good choices
Every day is an eternity
Each moment counts.

Our Journey

We have covered much ground together in our discussion of what it means to age actively and how to accomplish this objective. We want to emphasize that active aging is a journey, not a destination, and we continue to live and learn each day.

So, how did each of us face this journey as our lives were subjected to the research, writing, and talking with others about active aging? We are two different people—a couple with many years of collaboration in projects of this nature but with distinctive personalities and approaches to life, research, and writing. Here are reflections on the modeling of our lives while writing the book.

Barbara McCool

Did it work for me? Two years ago, my life mate and I decided to tackle a book about active aging systematically. We talked about the various dimensions of the topic, including physical, spiritual, emotional, intellectual, and social aspects of getting old. We then wrote in depth about each issue and evaluated our progress in each of these stated realms. One might imagine a months-long, intensive discussion about active aging. That would come close to our journey working on the transition to life in a retirement community while researching every aspect of our lives to guide our thinking about how to navigate our journey.

To provide a break from the transition, we went on a Caribbean Cruise. The cruise took place on a beautiful ship with a thousand other people, mostly strangers. The voyage during sunny skies and smooth waters was like manna from Heaven after a busy, challenging year of transition. Our Paradise in Arizona was a 4,000-square-foot house with a separate guesthouse on a four-acre oasis in the Sonoran Desert. Our residence now is a 1,500-square-foot, three-bedroom apartment in a retirement residence, in a densely populated urban area. This transition has been traumatic—going from freedom of movement in nature to tight spaces and more people than lived in our square-mile desert home.

One main takeaway from the cruise was the reality of older people on board the ship. Our life journey in coming from a community with a wide range of ages to a population of senior citizens mirrored this group. Many passengers used canes, some were in wheelchairs, and many relied on others for navigating the ship. Balancing this group was a smaller but vibrant number of couples and single adults engaged with life, carrying on stimulating conversations.

The most telling learning for me was that 20 percent or more of the ship's population was obese, some morbidly so. These individuals could barely walk, looked fatigued, and seemed dependent on another person to navigate the main ship events. Bottom line for me—I do not want to be part of this group as I add years to my life! Weight and many infirmities stem from inactivity and eating habits over which I have some control. Exerting that control is a responsibility that I need to take more seriously.

Our thesis is that you have to focus on the essential events of active aging and practice them each day.

Whether we stressed these key elements sufficiently or made a case for them will be judged by each reader. In summary, this is what I have learned so far in this examination process.

Physical Wellness

In the research for this book, I examined my eating habits to find ones that keep me vibrant and alive as I go about daily tasks. The big lessons learned are that I need to cut back on sugar and focus on eating more fish, lean meat, fibrous vegetables, and fruits. To accompany this regimen, I need to drink lots of water and eliminate snacks between meals.

I also need to get out of chairs and frequently move throughout the day. Exercise becomes my elixir of longevity. If I don't focus on locomotion, my muscles will atrophy, my bones will lose their strength, and my demeanor will be drab and vulnerable to disease attacks.

Daily walking routines, swimming, muscle strengthening, regular stretching, and dancing reduce my body mass index, clear my mind, and give me confidence that today is going to be useful in every way.

Emotional Wellness

Now that I am in the final years of life, I try each day to soften the rough edges of my personality, be more open to those around me who need love and attention, and accept the trials and sufferings necessary for my entrance into Heaven. Life is good: my goals are clear and straightforward, and I'm aware of what's going on in my reality; God is near!

Living in a faith-based retirement center has been excellent. The values that drive this particular community are the Christian principles of love and respect for others. Therefore attention to the presence of God and seeking guidance for action through the gospel and the biblical commandments guide my life.

I live with people who, in growing older, experience the physical, psychological, and spiritual assaults on their body, mind, and spirit. Their continual presence helps me see that I am on the far end of the birth-death continuum. My days are not unlimited, so I want to take advantage of this time to grow in grace and wisdom.

I gain strength from weekly Mass and discussion groups around problems in contemporary Christianity. We study issues such as gender identity, papal infallibility, gender definition for the priesthood, child abuse, nuclear proliferation, abortion and warring in weak countries, aggression by strong nations against the weak, and the terror tactics of the insecure against the strong. These issue help me see the Church as a vital force in solving today's complex social dilemmas.

My life at Bishop Spencer Place is excellent. I'm gradually adjusting to a more-organized lifestyle after the freedom and creativity of twenty years at Spirit Base Camp. Every day I'm aware that I have been created by a loving, all-knowing God who has formed me in His likeness and is getting me ready to join Him in Heaven forever.

My role in all of this is to grow in prayerfulness, ethical dealings with everyone, love, and serve those in need, and a constant awareness that God is working through me and directing my life.

I will strive to be authentic by being true to my values and principles that have evolved during my life of service. They include:

- **Being present for others, especially those suffering.** Moreover, be sure to include events that bring joy. Some situation are challenging, including being there for people in their loneliness and despair caused by mental and physical suffering.

- **Being honest.** Knowing who I am and remaining true to my core ideals. No one gains from self deception.

- **Listening to my heart; that deep, intuitive sense is essential to staying true to oneself.** I strive for a stance of kindness, peace, and deep mindfulness regarding everything that is happening. This mindfulness stance assumes a core centering that acknowledges a higher power that assists me in accepting my strengths and weaknesses. I use my intellectual, emotional, and physical gifts to understand and respond appropriately to people and situations. My priority in life is to engage in events that manifest heart and meaning.

- **Paying attention to the flow of events, gaining insights into the forces acting on outcomes, and then taking**

right action. Avoid early attachment to specific results, and seek understanding and common ground among competing ideas and ideals. I continually focus on my life goal–being united forever with my Creator and all the people I have known and loved in this life. In this journey of life, I intend to focus on a process that eliminates my rough edges and strengthens my love and compassion for everyone I meet.

Spiritual Wellness

I am a creature of God, placed in this world at this particular time so I can grow as a loving and compassionate person. As part of this lifetime commitment to God, I have focused on everything that happens to me as a vehicle for becoming the person I am intended to be. The special people in my life, the experiences—both good and bad—and the many encounters with the spiritual dimensions of living have been sent to me by a loving God. His plan for me is being worked out as I go about my daily life—as I undergo physical, mental, emotional, and spiritual trials, and as I grow closer to God through prayer and meditation.

Intellectual Wellness

Where would I be in life without a well-developed mind that can solve complex problems and find and accept new ways of living and assisting others? Continuing to learn is required to learn how to sort through new ideas, procedures, and methods relating to an ever-changing environment.

As I rid myself of old mindsets and performance habits, I find myself increasingly confident as I go into unfamiliar situations and quickly blend into the new environment. I welcome new ideas. Daily, I feed my mind with current events, new ways of thinking, and creative approaches to solving complex problems. When feasible, I try to engage in conversations that address world and local problems with old and new ways of managing intractable dilemmas. Some questions are never "solved" but must be managed to achieve workable peace.

I also seek learning opportunities. I look for lectures or meetings that explore areas of personal interest, or I talk with exciting people. I also try to invent creative approaches to troublesome problems. The bottom line in my learning is to keep my brain active so I can use this great gift to grow as a person and explore this beautiful world.

More importantly, doing this case study of our two-person experiment in how to age in a productive, healthy manner has brought back many of the theories and ideas for improving health care delivery. There are many avenues to pursue in reconnecting with earlier dreams of doing good work.

Social Wellness

Relationships and activities outside of my personal space expand my view of the world and increase my capacity for finding new friends and social situations. I seek ways to expand my comfort zone. I want to see and talk to people from other countries and participate in their family celebrations. I also engage in group discussions with others who have divergent opinions. Exposure to different cultures helps me function better in stressful situations while exposing quirks in my own stance toward the world.

The world is such an exciting place. My goal, until I die, is to learn as much as I can about all facets of this beautiful Planet Earth and its inhabitants.

Summing Up

Writing this book provided an excellent push for me to examine my life about myself, Monty, my immediate environment at Bishop Spencer Place, my relatives, good friends, professional colleagues, and the broad array of human beings I have yet to meet and will try to understand.

My world will shrink as I face the realities of getting older. However, my mind, spirit, and emotions can continue to grow and expand as I reach for the stars and prepare for everlasting life.

This book, which has forced me to do a great deal of research and writing, reminds me daily of the challenges to grow in the physical, emotional, spiritual, and social realms of living in our complicated culture. Following the principles for being in the present, having a life purpose, loving others, being guided by a Higher Power who monitors my steps as I navigate this modern life apprenticeship.

Monty Brown

We contemplated writing this book before we retired in Arizona, so the journey to age actively, in a healthy manner and to chronicle the journey began twenty-five or more years earlier. We did some writing about it then because it seemed important for the prevention of many chronic illnesses. We wrote about active aging in a few editorials but needed to live it first while we put down on paper the theory of what might work.

In 2014, I underwent heart surgery, nineteen years after retiring and lots of active living. I was working on recovery when we decided it was time to do the book. We had learned a lot, knew of many pitfalls, and had managed to survive it all. Now we were on our way to a new phase of life, one worth taking time to think through, research, and write about. In an authentic sense, the purpose of our study was to gather the latest thinking on all aspects of aging. We needed that knowledge base to fuel our thinking about how to live out our last years. Also, it was time to write a book on our life-guiding principle of active aging. Of course, we also wanted to be sure our last chapter fulfilled our desire to have our health span equal our life span.

My newly acquired habit of painting beckoned as well. It has always been my habit to work on more than one idea or project at a time. Art is one activity I now engage in, and research and active living are others. While painting delivers beauty, writing about active aging will reveal ideas we can share with others. Reading and study feed both.

I count one day at a time as a success. Beyond that is extra time that I plan to use living actively. If no new day arrives for me, that is within perfectly normal limits. At worst, the ideals of active aging are harmless. On the upside, life continues to be useful, as predicted. As we finish this book, I can also report that I've completed at least fifty new paintings as well. One day at a time doing what can be done each day is sufficient to accomplish goals.

Physical Wellness

My journey back to physical wellness began in earnest after heart surgery. It took at least six months. My strength and stamina were not back to pre-surgery for at least a year. My workouts have gone from thirty minutes to at least one hour every day. I also do high-intensity bursts to spice up walking, treadmill, and Nustep exercises.

Strength, stamina, balance, and more have become more explicitly scheduled. Here we can consult physical fitness professionals for advice on how to proceed. Most public health recommendations seem based on a judgment call that suggests less time will get more people to exercise with a hope that, once begun, they will do more.

Many simple things, such as walking stairs more often instead of using elevators, add to the daily exercise. More recently, I have used taken a short exercise break every hour to avoid complete inactivity for long periods.

Exercise keeps the body—including my brain, nervous system, and mind—working well. It does help with weight management, but what we eat makes the vast difference in our health. Many of the "low fat, bad fats, some fats" messages from health officials have probably done us more harm than good. But something worked; we're still here.

Regarding my weight management, changes in eating habits first included a calorie count with lots of fish and vegetables and eliminating most desserts and bread from meals. After a lot more study and experimentation with approaches, I opted for two meals a day, with a fast from after dinner to lunch the following day about fifteen hours later. I am refreshed in the morning and have one and sometimes two coffees (one of them decaf) before lunch with whole milk, so technically it's not a full fifteen-hour fast. As of this writing, I do a daily eighteen-hour fast, thus eating my daily food allowance in a six-hour, and often shorter, window of time. More recently, I have fasted thirty hours without any problems and with a slight weight loss, one I had needed after being stuck at the same weight for a time.

I have also used a two-day routine: one day with a fourteen-hour fast and two meals, and the second day with a twenty-hour fast and one main meal. It is much easier to stay on a reduced- calorie diet in this manner. For most days, calorie counting isn't necessary; limiting which foods I eat and eating only two meals a day keeps my weight either steady or at a slow decline.

This eating schedule gives me a good start on reading, writing, and daily exercise before my first meal of the day. At that meal, I eat four hundred to five hundred calories and maybe drink another decaf coffee. Dinner for us is around 5:30 p.m. I have no hunger issues, drink lots of water, and read, write, or paint during the other hours. So, on most days, I eat around a fifteen-hundred-calorie diet, with lots of greens in one meal and fish or meat plus veggies in another. Desserts have only a tiny place in my life now.

Producing this book was, for me, like winning a lottery. The research and writing were absorbing and led to many changes in my approach to exercise and eating, resulting in a healthier lifestyle. Fitness, weight management, and intellectual engagement top my list of things most helpful to staying active as I age.

Emotional Wellness

Meditation and the more contemplative ideas are areas of interest for me. Many readings focus on reducing stress. Being by nature somewhat introverted, I tend toward a degree of calmness that is further guided by the ideas of getting rid of negative emotions against others. It also helps to remember that we often cannot change the external stressors or the opinions of others, but we can and should manage how we react to them. Many ideas in the meditation, mindfulness, and consciousness literature speak to such issues.

Relaxation techniques can help deal with health and emotionally laden events of life. However, my approach to calmness and flow is to move over to painting, or, from time to time, write a poem to go with a sketch. Stillness from a meditative practice is not a method I have adopted. Quiet, allowing my mind to engage with color or flow with words, is more the style I follow. Listening to music with hooded eyes can be moving for the energy fields present in my being.

One of life's significant stressors is that many good intentions and goals are never realized. There are ways to handle this kind of problem. I try to review what I want to accomplish each day; each morning I think about the day, how it is likely to go, and what I will do regarding my current goals. For instance, I have eating goals and methods for achieving them. Making things specific to the day also applies to physical activities. Indeed, a morning review is something we often do as a couple. Many current aging goals can become habits more quickly by doing them with another person. Daily reports and goal setting works well for me.

Insights from writing and research morphed into a life-redesign project. We have made many life redesign plans with good results. However none have been with such intentionality and such depth of research and experimentation. This stage of life is one in which we will transposition from vibrant, independent, self-directed living to a life with increased support, and dependency. However, by doing this book and life redesign, it is our intention not to forget to live fully, actively, and independently to that ultimate end.

Much of my emotional balance comes from engaging in the work of painting, writing, reading, and communicating. In this way of living, I focus on being in the present, and my attention is on what is happening right now. Negative thoughts are relatively easy to banish through direct action when possible, or through other means discussed in the book.

Those of us in this community are brought together in part by the fact that everyone has a chronic condition that needs attention; we all share the status of aging to the near edge of the human life span. Aging itself is the chronic condition needing treatment, and we are each our own best caregiver. More opportunities exist in retirement communitiesN to acknowledge and greet one another, to interact with many people daily who need social support. Socializing is now a major daily life event.

Spiritual Wellness

My religious beliefs were shaped early on by Christian values, although formal teachings about such values and church attendance were mostly absent. Over the years, I adopted many of the teachings of Jesus and others, with little systematic cataloging of the origins of different ideas. My sense of creation comes from reading about the universe(s), consciousness writings, and my knowledge that we have a purpose in our lives. No doubt Buddhism has taken root for me as well. No doubt other customs and habits have accreted along the way as well. So be it, we are a culture of cultures in the US, so too in our genetic makeup.

Even if there is no ultimate Creator, purpose in life by choice greatly enriches my days. My ultimate goal tends toward service to others, kindness, and action. In public health, the idea is to improve the health of people, which fits my sense of a grand purpose in life. Also, health care provides intellectual challenges, accomplished people, and a strong work ethic. My sense of purpose is coupled with a career dedicated to improving the lives of others; life doesn't get much better than that.

My early thoughts about a focus for life in work or significant pursuits were more about satisfying simple goals, such as earning money necessary to buy a comic book or go to the weekly movies to enjoy the thrill of seeing Tarzan swing through the trees. Along the way many of the preachers and evangelist and aspirational writers left the mark on my psychological make up including Norman Vincent Peal, Billy Graham, and others who urge one to aspire to greater things, to live a positive life, to think positive thoughts. I was primed early to hear the message of psychology thought leaders Maslow and Rogers. Later, not having any specific occupation in mind, my focus shifted to improving and expanding personal knowledge and skills to be ready for opportunities that might arise. This sense of purpose still drives much of my life. I love the idea of growth and learning and exercising the mind, and, increasingly, using the body. Moreover, for me, it is and always was body-mind-spirit connected to all energy fields, all the time. The shifts in matter and form occur, but the essence is forever.

The foundation of my daily community goal is to look out for someone needing a boost. Although my personality is mostly introverted, my humor tends toward the personal, and I use it to boost those around me. Using humor fits with one of the essential guidelines presented here. Acting in the present and on problems and issues in front of us serves us and others. A little humor goes a long way toward giving others an energy boost. It is a bit harder for me to initiate conversation. I do it when it seems to help, and, in a life of teaching, consulting, and other work, it has been necessary to master acts more appropriate to more extroverted personality types.

During these months of research and writing, my sense of the divine in all grows. It is not a stretch for me to sense a Creator for these complex energy fields. We are a part of those fields, and it would not surprise me that once our parents connect the genetic mapping begins. Over time more learning, growing and accretion occurs. Each of us has at every stage of life choices of direction make. Of course when young those choices are made for us. As we reach high school, it is up to each of us to make the most of what we have. I accept the idea that our eternal existence is part and parcel of how the system works and that all forms change over time. Others can help but the big decisions we each make more or less on our own.

In a genuine sense to me, Jesus and the Holy Spirit are right here all the time, guiding my steps, but whether that is more than a metaphor than any physical reality matters less to me than how guidance from these teachings has influenced my life. Whatever the ultimate truth might be, it is incredible to be alive, to live a day at a time, to enjoy this journey of life.

Things were good before this current project, but my life has deepened because of it. Redesigning life for active aging and redoing ones lifestyle on occasion works exceptionally well for me. In a very real sense, each day present opportunities to shift directions. Habits take longer to set but every day one can begin a new direction. Not every pathway may be open but so far at 88 many choices are still available.

Intellectual Wellness

The other subjects in this book were beneficial for me, but the intellectual stimulation of researching the working of the brain, the connections among the mind, physical, emotional, spiritual, and other factors was and remains a feast. My brain function improved throughout writing this book. It would not surprise me to learn at some point that brain function declined as a result of stress during cardiac surgery. Nor would

I be surprised if it could be proved that my changes in exercise and diet have been improving brain functioning. It is rational to think that improvement has occurred and that our work pays real dividends.

One of our concerns as we age is avoiding or mitigating Alzheimer's disease. I assess that the more one can stimulate the brain and keep learning new things, the more likely one is to vitalize the mind. Education, reading, mental stimulation, and more are encouraged by many. As former academics who took more degrees than needed for our work and who routinely go on vacations to learn new things, intellectual stimulation is a significant passion. In addition, I also believe that eliminating lots of sugar from my diet and getting more healthy fats and fiber all have had a positive impact on my brain functioning.

I am a big user of computers and engage in writing commentary on many subjects. One concern I have about this is that keeping a focus on essential matters is too easily distracted by emails, little bells ringing, ads popping up when reading an article online, and more.

I now realize how much my itch to learn is about things related to influences on my life. I do not remember a time when I was not curious about something. When my earnings were merely a few dollars a week, I bought every new comic book of interest. I read them and then gave them away. No doubt those books fueled my incessant desire to explore and learn.

**We can change course today,
We can act today on our environment,
We may modify what started yesterday;
But for life, it is one day at a time.**

We can mentally think about tomorrow, we can anticipate the needs of tomorrow, but today, only in the present can we act on our intentions. Tomorrow will benefit from the learning and problem identification done today which can, perhaps, be applied to the present on that days as it dawns. How? Dream time, dream time.

Dreams can clarify, amply, eliminate or as often happens, change the nature of the problem and potential solutions. Nighttime mental processing often delivers excellent ideas. Indeed learning how to have more vivid dreams and knowingly participate in the dreams is a new opportunity for intellectual growth. Imagine how much more productive we can be if instead of the 15 or so waking hours for work and learning, we can add another 4-8 hours more! While I have done it for years it has recently become of more interest and usefulness. Dream time is not limited to the more mundane activities of daily living, but more often become the pivot point for more critical issues including how to approach a next painting or poem.

If our action is limited to the present, it makes logical sense to review life goals (all goals, really) and each day give thought to what can be done to move toward those goals. In my exercise and focus on weight management, daily reviews have greatly improved my results. Weight loss of forty pounds held for over a year now is positive proof to support the methods I've chosen. We can not only find ways that offer delicious eating but also at the same time choose options that achieve good results. Daily reviewing the things before us results in much more efficient use of our time, more fun, and more comfortable goal accomplishment. Reading, writing, and explicit thought to designing my life is a result of this work, and this book is a byproduct of such. But these are not the only growth tools at our disposal; I remind the reader that dream time works with knowledge and all else recorded to date for its possible use in the present, which today we call tomorrow. Life is not only the time of our being awake as we know it; growth is continuous and has no limits until we cease to exist.

Social Wellness

As I write this, I am dressed for a party; I'm going out shortly to connect and socialize. Even an introvert like me enjoys one of life's greatest gifts—the companionship of people. We all need it. I get more here in apartment living with shared dining and other activities. It is suitable for me, and it also provides daily opportunities to help others, another gift we have. The more we help others, the better we tend to feel about ourselves.

We make and aid new friendship developments in many ways. Socializing helps cement relations while exercising; one can meet others while dining, and bonding is facilitated with just plain talk while on elevators or walking in hallways or waiting in line for service. We have also noted other opportunities to create conditions for more socializing. For me, it is especially helpful to find others who like to dig deeper into issues without getting hung up on political talking points. We have seen other ideas that we can fit into the routines here that have benefitted us and will benefit our neighbors. It is amazing the many ways in which these group settings can be of assistance in meeting our collective needs for socialization.

No doubt the book has heightened my awareness of the need to stay socially connected. Our life designs are taking us in the direction of more of it. It is easy to find ways to get into groups doing things of interest.

We heartily recommend more socializing. Life is cruel in one significant way; over time, friends and neighbors pass away, so having new friends is always a good idea. Finding a few with whom one can share the more intimate details of life is even more critical. These are the things we dedicate much of our work to accomplish. It works for us, and we recommend it to others.

This journey into life design for active aging has been much hard work, much fun, and contributed to many lifestyle adjustments for each of us. The work has begun, and it will unfold in the years just ahead. No doubt the search for meaning in this life will continue. The journey goes on until it reaches life's event horizon.

Other Thoughts

Looking back on writing this book, I realize that it reasonably describes how my life progresses. Life is an ongoing quest to see what is out there. I am from a poor family living in a small mill town in the middle of a state-designed pine forest, and what was outside that isolated town stimulated a passionate life of learning. At an early age, I asked around town for jobs and found one. Pay for work bought comic books that were mostly science fiction; these books served for many years as my personal reading. Science fiction transported me into beautiful worlds that were inspirational for a questing mind. Work was more for income than the inherent interest in the work, but every job had exciting things to learn. Resources for learning was a driving force.

In retirement, that interest continues, and I now focus often on what it takes to live a healthy life. What is life? Science fiction is no longer favored go-to reading for me. Science itself offers clues, hypothesis, potential prescriptions, and things to try. Overall, however, my reading practice hasn't changed; it remains an exploration, a search for meaning, a glimpse around the bend and over the next hill.

I believe that one purpose of living is to explore our environment to ascertain how it works. Active aging works for me. Why? The search goes on, and insight is growing out of science. Some of who I am is a result of the genes I've inherited. Other parts of me have developed through interaction with the world around me. A war came just as I finished high school; the Air Force years brought testing, schooling, growth, opportunity to interact with college graduates, and, eventually, college and a world of ideas to explore.

Life beyond ones genes is shaped by happy accidents. One of the blessings for me is that I have taken advantage of many such happy accidents. Being aware of the potential in those accidents is itself probably a heritable trait. On the other hand many of the aspirational writers make a big point about looking all events for their life lessons. But for those heritable traits, life might have been very different. However, for me, life has been on big opportunity and filled with happy accidents. Little has taken away from this fact. It matter not to me that others were born to royalty, some to inherited riches, and still others attended the most renowned of schools. I live free and with great opportunity for improvement. No one has more than those who seize the day and move forward.

CHAPTER TEN (Q&A)

1. After writing this book, what are the takeaways that stay with you?

The biggest is the realization that today I have a whole new basket of learning opportunities arising from this work. With the completion of the book its meaning propels us to move out and extoll its message for other to use. The writing has humble us to realize how much we still have to learn on so many levels.

Then there are the learnings from the studies of Active Aging. How will I keep my weight down now that our meals are now catered, with choices but with a limited selection of ingredients? How will I battle using food as an antidote to small stresses that occur routinely in congregate living conditions?

How can we continually dedicate our time and energy to making the right choices in eating, exercising, working with others, and relating to God in positive ways? What techniques will we use to maintain enthusiasm for this new path of wellness and wholeness?

Finally, are we getting ready for our Death? Death is an inevitable reality. Will we have the will and patience to surrender to the direction of others who will care for us in the final days and who will usher us into the other life?

So what is the big take away? We know little that can be said and yet all of life is remarkably similar. We are here in the present and can enjoy the study of our being here. We can try to use our given talents and opportunities to live a fuller life and be useful to others. We come away with more questions than answers.

2. Did things you studied and learned have noticeable impacts on your behavior?

Without a doubt, things that we read, study, and write about become, to some degree, part of us and our behavior. Exercising was not a big part of our life before the book, but now it's a well-established practice, and with improvements as well. We are dedicated readers of all new reports on how to do better at it. High-intensity interval training, while not a new idea to us, has become gospel for Monty. When his weight goes back up a bit, he tackles it quickly with tools we now incorporate into our routines. Weight issues remain a challenge for both of us.

Both of us have sought and lobbied our retirement home for a variety of exercise classes such as Tai Chi, yoga, swimming, strength training, and routine walking pathways. Many of these needed programs now exist, and residents are participating. Discussions about growth in fitness, balance, and mindfulness come up often.

Many of our eating behaviors have changed: We do some fasting routinely. We find ways to get more fiber into our diet. And we also eat more salads.

3. Were there any changes that surprised you?

Some things were unexpected. Early in the move to try to get the diet right, Monty decided to go off of Prilosec and later told his physician. He had become leery of its impact on nutrient extraction. He doesn't recall any one thing that prompted that action. New eating habits have corrected the problem; GERDS is no longer an issue for him. We don't recommend doing this without physician consultation; he did eventually consult a physician, who endorsed the practice. Caution: we do often change things before consulting a physician but not before our research has allowed us to make a considered judgment on an issue. It would be best to become informed, ask, and then take action.

4. **When you finished writing this book, were there subjects not yet fully explored? Are there any topics that might receive more of your attention later?**

Yes, to both questions. First, the right way to diet for losing weight and which foods are ideal for one to consume remains controversial, as we have noted. However, there are elements of books we've read, whose insights are shared here, which we continue to learn from as we explore the subject on an ongoing basis. In short, this is a journey begun, not finished, nor the secrets to assured success revealed. One area Monty is exploring now is the use of supplemental nutrients. We know how many vitamins and minerals are leached from the soil by monoculture and overuse of the earth and how our genetic modification of plants and livestock is resulting in multiple changes that are concerning to scientists and consumers. Moreover, we have, from time to time, adopted the use of some supplements. However, we have not paid close attention to the ingredients even of the things we use. This research has made us better consumers of information.

5. **Are there some areas of research you believe hold promise for making it more likely that individual consumers can be more informed about what they need to do to improve their health while aging?**

We are exploring several areas of research that offer greater insight. Sleep is far more important than we had thought. Sleep, a phase of our daily lives, takes up a third of our day. We have long thought that one needed to get about eight hours of restful sleep nightly to function well. Since reading more about it and using more of the advice on getting good sleep—eight or more hours a night OF

HIGH QUALITY SLEEP is a major goal. Now our 8 hours has gone a bit longer and some other changes have improve sleep quality. As in other areas, much is still unknown about what is true, but what is already known may be more important than other subjects that are being given much more attention.

Genetic testing will play a significant role in the future of medicine. Enough is known for this to already play a vital role in some areas, even in the field of prevention and counseling regarding approaches to subjects covered in this book. Topics like metabolism, oxidative stress, and nutritional supplements are complicated. Dealing with such issues needs more attention; our personal approach is to research, consult, and practice to see what fits for us.

6. **Is this book more of a personal journey about your life design project, or is it something that is meant to provide things others can do?**

It is primarily a personal life design project. The idea of active aging is also a professionally recommended goal for people to do. Each person must, of course, design their path. Each path has different gifts and flaws. Not everything works for everyone; each person needs to work through and find what works for them. So, it is a personal journey but one filled with insights from our evaluation and use of the many sources available to those interested in this kind of adventure.

7. **There is more information available today about the importance of having a life purpose. Purpose often refers to something beyond one's self. Can you elaborate on your life purpose and how it relates to something other than yourself being healthy?**

Throughout this personal journey, this has been a constant question. Are we doing this for us, or is it for others? If just for us that would seem to be a bit narcissistic. If for others, how would it manifest our life purpose? We are retired, and most of the help and advice we get asked for or offer is for friends, neighbors, and family. Our writing is not widely published anymore, and artwork mainly adorns our walls and any available space in our small retirement apartment.

While this research and writing will reach only a few, it has another more important purpose. We endorse the belief that one should do unto others what one would have others do unto them. The Golden Rule is a two-pronged test. One must know what is best for oneself in order to make an informed decision on what would be best for others. If one is to take care of a family when they are in distress, one must be capable first of having the strength, wisdom, and means to care for oneself. Active aging is far more critical as one reaches an older age. Aging people must depend upon themselves to make important next-step decisions. It is important to remain independent so as not to burden others. It is also essential to be healthy and alert if one is to be of help to another. Our life's purpose of caring for one another is as strong as ever, and the time of need for such strength and wisdom is even more critical.

The Golden rule admonishes us to understand what would help us so that we might do as much for another. Our advice is to study the studies and stories of others and try their suggestions to see how they work for you. Life is a one-person journey, and not anything seems to be ideally suited for everyone. So study to live actively and do what works for you.

8. Any last thoughts?

You can act today to change your life. Physical exercise, mental training, and challenging yourself to do better can improve your experience at any age. Working the body helps the mind, and cognitive training improves total functioning. It is all about being active. Serve others, be generous; good deeds are food for life and living. Keep moving.

9. What happens next with this book?

That is a good question. When we retired from active consulting and moved to Tucson, we began a life devoted more to being close to the community in which we lived. Our academic and consulting lives were devoted mostly to our profession and knew no regional boundaries; the practice was national. In our Tucson retirement, our activities were limited mostly to our neighborhood and its neighboring Saguaro National Park. With the 9/11/2001 terror attacks and resultant national mobilization, we took on major volunteer regional, and some state, roles. Since moving to Kansas City, our work has been devoted to a life design review and writing about it as well as Active Aging designs to improve health. So now, what comes next?

We will self-publish the book in sufficient copies to share it with professional colleagues who are still in active career roles. What happens next depends on whether anyone or any agency finds it of sufficient interest to publish it and distribute it more broadly. Our aging journey is not sufficiently active to mount another career effort to take these ideas to a broader audience. We have been there, done that, and have neither the energy nor desire to do it again. We have other gifts to share, so this book goes on the wind for possible use. We go on to other interests, including sharing this with others in close proximity to our current home territory. We go on to Active Aging. We make travel plans for next year. We fully engage with the authorship and marketing of the book. Painting and marketing efforts pick up. We are active agers.

We hope that this book is useful to others.

—Barbara McCool and Montague Brown

ABOUT THE AUTHORS

Is this book reflective of the state of the science on the issues, or about just a couple of people, or, perhaps, some combination of both? Environment and history no doubt influence how we live. The science, while not settled in most areas of concern, definitely points in the direction of staying active to mitigate the ravages of old age and chronic diseases. At the same time, individuals differ significantly in how they use information. Much of this writing reflects a personal journey that flows from a history of the search for knowledge and pushing limits. Throughout the book, we've used our experiences to illustrate significant points.

Barbara McCool
RN, BA, MHA, MTP, and PhD

Now in her eighties and living at Bishop Spencer Place, a Continuing Care Community in Kansas City, Missouri, Barbara is a health care professional serving for fifty years as a clinician, hospital administrator, educator, researcher, and consultant. Grounded in the Midwestern values of being a strong Christian and serving others, she has systematically developed the skills to be a leader in health care. She accomplished her goals.

Barbara has worked in hospitals, clinics, universities, government agencies, and private industries and held faculty appointments at Ohio State, Northwestern, Duke, and Kansas universities. For eighteen years, she served as a member of the Sisters of Charity of Leavenworth, a religious congregation of women who owned and managed hospitals and schools throughout the United States. In this, she grounded herself in the Christian values of love and service to others.

During those years of service in a religious congregation, she became a nurse, worked in many settings, finished her registered nurse training and later a bachelors degree and hospital administration degree. She worked across the country, stoked boilers at times, aided in delivering babies, and ran hospital operations. She eagerly sought learning opportunities at each stop along the way as she moved up in her chosen and assigned service duties. After leaving the Sisters of Charity of Leavenworth, she began a teaching career and secured grants to pursue and complete a doctorate leading to a university career. In each post, she contributed to research programs and pioneered new programs.

Barbara has published many articles and four books. She was an associate editor of *Health Care Management Review* and served on several boards of national health care systems and health-related task forces. Her professional focus was on building vertically integrated health care systems and the development of high-performing health care executives.

She earned her baccalaureate degree from the University of Saint Mary in Leavenworth, Kansas; her master of heath administration from the University of Minnesota; her doctoral degree in Education from Ohio State University; and her master's in transpersonal psychology from the Institute of Transpersonal Psychology in Menlo Park, California. In her professional education, she engaged in a lifelong effort to improve her intellectual, social, and spiritual skills and performance to serve people.

Married to Monty Brown for forty-six years, Barbara combined her skills with Monty to develop a new professional practice in the development of vertically integrated health care systems through consulting, teaching, writing, and speaking. Their time as a couple focuses on growth in healthy living, spirituality, intellectual acumen, creative arts, beautiful living sites, time with family and friends, and a commitment to "Grow or Die."

This book is the culmination of a long journey in staying alive and being open to every possibility to become a fully functioning active ager! Writing the book represents the basis for another stage of life. Now, as it is being finished, another chapter of life is beginning.

Montague (Monty) Brown
AB, MBA, DrPH, JD

Monty was born in 1931, in Whitmire, South Carolina, a cotton mill town, to William B. and Minnie Vaughn Brown, both with little education and jobs in a cotton mill. In 1949, the family moved to Great Falls, South Carolina, another cotton mill town, where Monty took his mill job as a weaver(he had a lesser skilled job in Whitmire) and, later, apprenticed as a loom mechanic. Monty dropped out of school but returned the next year when his parents moved to North Carolina. With his return to finish high school and his family moving to a new town and jobs,he made his new home in aa bed and breakfast boarding house. He worked a full time cotton mill job, forty-hour-per-week, on evening shifts. This was a seminal year for Monty. The boarding house was mainly populated with school teachers and visiting mill executives, all college graduates, a class of people heretofore unknown to him. At school he was elected class president and later at graduation time, he was one of the main speakers. From these exposures college became a budding dream.

In 1950, Monty graduated high school and joined the US Air Force to serve in the Korean War. First an enlisted man who moved from an air police job, to a cook squadron but diverted to a clerks position before being trained as a radar mechanic. He later became an aircraft observer. During his five-plus years of active service, he spent nearly three years mostly in electronics and aircraft observer training. Systems paradigms widely used in electronics were invaluable as his later training was only beginning to use this model of thinking. He left active duty as a First Lieutenant. In the reserves, he left service three or so years later as a

Captain. Monty' aspirations for more education was greatly accelerated in the military. His test scores got him into high quality technical training. And in those classes he successfully competed with college graduates. In a way he began to see that he could do this as well. Being in Texas, he applied to the University of Texas; and knowing California to have great universities he applied to U. C. Berkley. And with his home in South Carolina he applied there as well. All granted admission with up to 2 years of advanced credits for prior experience. He also applied to the University of Chicago which admitted him but with any credits to depend on testing to ascertain how well he did compared to their graduates. He chose U.Chicago in part because of their strong liberal arts undergraduate program and what he considered the most rational approach to granting credits. Because of the testing and his choice of graduate school, he began graduate courses his second year at UC and got an AB just two quarter before an MBA. He love affair with learning grew by leaps and bounds.

In 1955, Monty began his college education at the University of Chicago, Illinois, where he received both a bachelors degree and masters in business administration and completed sufficient course work for a doctoral degree in business. While there, he married and fathered three daughters. In addition to his college course work, he worked odd service jobs and served as a research assistant to three different professors and Assistant Dean of Students in the business school. While Monty was a student he did a study of a union strike near his home. After that work well for his, he immersed himself in hospital human resources and labor relations studies by taking courses across the university. That study led to publications, doctoral programs, fellowships, and more. Part of his academic journey took him to the Industrial Relations Institute, where he developed attitude surveys for hospital workers, doctors, and patients. He spoke at dozens of meetings of hospital executives in over thirty states on the subject of labor relations. All of this led to full-time engagement in the hospital administration field.

This speech making led to greater knowledge of the healthcare field and more research opportunities along with fellowship and research funding. Monty's penchant for following his own muse led to many engaged and interesting explorations of health care management but it did not make him a good student. After an assessment by a psychologist, he was told, your aptitudes would make you a great psychiatrist but you would flunk medical school, if things aren't of interest you have too little patience to master them.

Upon leaving the university to manage a research and development arm of the New Jersey Hospital Association, Monty obtained grants and managed an effort to establish training programs for nurses' aides and other hospital workers. While getting research and development grants for such applications, he acquired a fellowship that included salary replacement, tuition, and other expenses to get a doctorate to direct educational programs for hospital administrators.

That fellowship led to a doctor of public health, DrPH, degree majoring in health administration. From there he became an associate professor and Director of a Health Administration Program in the Kellogg School of Management. During that time, he became divorced and later married Barbara McCool. They were both offered sabbaticals at the National Center for Health Services Research and professorships at Duke University. During that sabbatical year, Monty wrote a book on multi-hospital systems, which placed him in front of a development that is still playing out—consolidation in health care delivery systems. While at Duke, Monty became editor of *Health Care Management Review* and held that post for twenty-five years or so. It provided a full window on the field of practice, a wonderful outlet for his ideas, and insights into the best thinkers in the field.

His research and writing on multi-hospital systems and mergers entailed frequent contacts with legal issues and lawyers. After moving to Duke University, he decided to pursue the study of law rather than do more direct economic or organizational research of systems. This switch was related the field he was already in since he considered the law to have a significant impact on what hospitals can and cannot do and how they are organized.

After Monty finished law school, Barbara needed to spend more time to support her widowed mother. Since Monty had not yet chosen between job opportunities in Chicago, New York City, and Washington, DC, he and Barbara moved to Kansas City where they developed a consulting practice. Over their decade of consulting, one of the ideas they explored was Active Aging. With retirement, that exploration expanded into life practices, and now with this research and writing it has become a lifetime practice for both of Monty and Barbara.

SUGGESTED READINGS

Since our early studies in public health, we've been attracted to the concept of prevention via lifestyle methods and have made it a subject of study, casual reading, and trying ideas. We have read and often personally tested theories, and suggestions garnered from thousands of articles, books, videos, and more. The titles below are some of the books we've recently read— some old, some new, and all containing useful and insightful views on the subjects covered in this book. We offer these as a token beginning to plumb the ideas of this book. Every author featured here offers windows on worlds of research and practice beyond the volumes. Besides, most if not all of these authors are found on YouTube videos, sometimes in lectures, sometimes interviews. We suggest you sample their thinking on other venues as well. Each offers nuances not offered by others. While some disagreement on issues appears, more in-depth reading listening can explain much about such appearances and the reasons for their differences. Much is known, much more remains opaque to science, and us.

Amen, Daniel G. (2015). *Change Your Brain, Change Your Life: The Breakthrough Program for Conquering Anxiety, Depression, Obsessiveness, Lack of Focus, Anger, Memory Problems.* New York: Harmony Books.

Ardell, Donald B. (1986). *High Level Wellness: An Alternative to Doctors, Drugs and Disease.* Berkeley: Ten Speed Press.

Arrien, Angeles. (2005). *The Second Half of Life: Opening the Eight Gates of Wisdom.* Boulder: Sounds True.

Arrien, Angeles. (1993). *The Four-Fold Way: Walking the Path of the Warrior, Teacher, Healer and Visionary.* San Francisco: Harper Collins.

Bredesen, Dale E. (2017). *The End of Alzheimer's: The First Program to Prevent and Reverse Cognitive Decline.* New York: Penguin Random House Group.

Briley, Julie & Jackson, Courtney. (2016). *Food as Medicine Everyday: Reclaim Your Health With Whole Foods.* Portland: NCNM Press.

Brooks, David. (2019). *The Second Mountain: The Quest for a Moral Life.* New York: Random House.

Brown, Bernie. (2018). *Dare to Lead: Brave Work, Tough Conversations, Whole Hearts.* London: Penguin Random House U.K.

Burnett, Bill & Evans, Dave. (2016). *Designing Your Life: How to Build a Well-Lived, Joyous Life.* New York: Alfred A Knopf.

Cameron, Julia. (2016). *The Artist's Way: A Spiritual Path to Higher Creativity.* New York: Penguin Random House Group.

Campbell, T. & Colin & Campbell II & Thomas M. (2017). *The China Study: The Most Comprehensive Study of Nutrition Ever Conducted and Startling Implications for Diet, Weight Loss and Long Term Health.* Dallas: Ben Bella Books.

Chodron, Pema (2001). *The Places That Scare You: A Guide to Fearlessness in Difficult Times.* Boston: Shambala.

Chodron, Pema (2013). *Living Beautifully.* Boulder: Shambala.

Csikszentmihalyi, Mihaly. (1990). *Flow: The Psychology of Optimal Experience.* New York: Harper Collins Publishers.

Dinicolantonio, James & Fung, Jason. (2019). *The Longevity Solution: Rediscovering Centuries Old Secrets to a Healthy, Long Life.* Las Vegas: Victory Belt Publishing.

Davidson, Alan. (2014). *Social Determinants of Health: A Comparative Approach.* Ontario: Oxford University Press.

Feldman, Christina. (2006). *The Buddhist Path to Simplicity: Spiritual Practice for Everyday Life.* New York: Barnes and Noble.

Feldman, Christina. (2005). *Compassion: Listening to the Cries of the World.* Boulder: Shambala.

Freudenberg, Nicholas. (2016). *Lethal But Legal: Corporations, Consumption and Protecting Public Health.* New York: Oxford University Press.

Fung, Jason. (2016). *The Obesity Code: Unlocking the Secrets of Weight Loss.* Berkeley: Greystone Books.

Fung, Jason. (2018). *The Diabetes Code: Unlocking the Secrets of Weigh Loss.*Berkeley: Greystone Books.

Gibala, Martin. (2017). *The One Minute Workout: Science Shows a Way to Get Fit That's Smarter, Faster, Shorter.* New York: Penguin Random House Group.

Gundry, Steven (2017). T*he Plant Paradox: The Hidden Dangers in "Healthy" Foods That Cause Disease and Weight Gain.* New York: Harper Collins.

Gundry, Steven (2019). *The Longevity Paradox: How to Die Young at a Ripe Old Age.* New York: Harper Collins.

Kabat-Zinn. Jon. (2012). *Mindfulness for Beginners: Reclaiming the Present Moment and Your Life.* Boulder: Sounds True.

Kaplan, Robert M. (2019). *More than Medicine: The Broken Promise of American Health.* Cambridge: Harvard University Press.

Knight, Rob. (2015). *Follow Your Gut: The Enormous Impact of Tiny Microbes.* New York: Simon & Schuster.

Kornfield, Jack. (2008). *Meditation for Beginners: Guided Meditation for Insight, Inner Clarity and Cultivating a Compassionate Heart.* Boulder: Sounds True.

Land, George TL. (1987) . *Grow or Die: The Unifying Principle of Transformation Revised Edition.* New Jersey: John Wiley & Sons.

Li, William W. (2019). *Eat to Beat Disease: The Body's Five Defense Systems and the Foods That Could Save Your Life.* New York: Grand Central Life and Style.

Ludwig, David. (2016). *Always Hungry: Conquer Cravings, Retrain Your Food Cells and Lose Weight Permanently.* New York: Penguin Random House Group.

Macy, Beth. (2018). *Dopesick: Dealers, Doctors and the Drug Company that Addicted America.* New York: Little, Brown and Company.

Mayo Clinic Staff. (2010). T*he Mayo Clinic Diet: Eat Well, Enjoy Life, Lose Weight.* Intercourse, PA: Good Books.

Mayo Clinic Staff. (2013). *Mayo Clinic on Healthy Aging: How to Find Happiness and Vitality for a Lifetime.* Rochester: Mayo Clinic Publishing.

Hensrud, Donald D. (2017). *The Mayo Clinic Diet Journal - 2nd Edition.* Rochester: Mayo Clinic Publishing.

McLaren, Karla. (2013). *The Art of Empathy: Complete Guide to Life's Most Essential Skill.* Boulder: Sounds True.

Mercola, Joseph. (2017). *Fat for Fuel: A Revolutionary Diet to Combat Cancer, Boost Brain Power and Increase Your Energy - 2nd Edition.* New York: Hay House.

O'Keefe, James and O'Keefe, Joan. (2013). *Let Me Tell You a Story: Inspirational Stories for Health, Happiness and a Sexy Waist.* Kansas City: Andrews McMeel Publishing.

Ornish, Dean and Ornish, Anne. (2019). *UnDo It!: How Simple Lifestyle Changes Can Reverse Most Chronic Diseases.* New York: Penguin Random House Group.

Parker, Riya. (2018). *The Art of Gathering: How We Meet and Why It Matters.* New York: Riverhead Books

Perlmutter, David (2018). *Grain Brain: The Surprising Truth About Wheat, Carbs and Sugar - Your Brain's Silent Killer*. New York: Little Brown Sparks.

Pinker, Steven (2018). *Enlightenment Now: The Case for Reason, Science, Humanism and Progress*. New York: Viking Press.

Ratcliff, Kathryn Strother (2017). *The Social Determinants of Health: Looking Upstream*. Cambridge: Polity Press.

Rogers, Carl (1961). *On Becoming a Person: A Therapist's View of Psychotherapy*. Boston: Houghton Mifflin Company

Rohr, Richard. (2003). *Everything Belongs: The Gift of Contemplative Prayer*. New York: Crossroads Publishing Company.

Salzberg, Sharon (2010). *The Force of Kindness: Change Your Life With Love and Compassion*. Boulder: Sounds True.

Smith, Paul R. (2011). *Integral Christianity: The Spirit's Call to Evolve*. St. Paul: Paragon House.

Sood, Amit (2013). *The Mayo Clinic Guide to Stress-Free Living*. Philadelphia: Perseus Book Group.

Travis, John and Ryan, Regina (2004). *Wellness Workbook: How to Achieve Enduring Health and Vitality*. Berkeley: Random House.

Villodo, Alberto (2019). *Grow a New Body*. New York: Hay House.

Walker, Matthew (2017). *Why We Sleep*. New York: Simon and Schuster.

Weber, Robert and Orsborn, Carol. (2015). *The Spirituality of Age: A Seeker's Guide to Growing Older*. Rochester: Park Street Press.

Weil, Andrew. (2007). *Healthy Aging: A Life-Long Guide to Your Well Being*. New York: Anchor Books

Wigglesworth, Cindy. (2012). *The Twenty-One Skills of Spiritual Intelligence*. New York: Select Books.